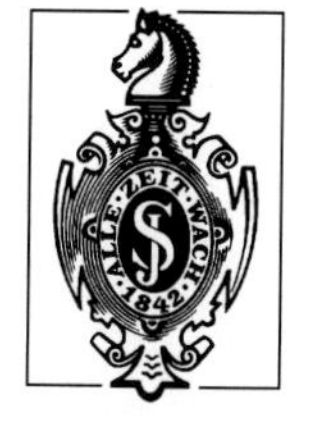

Klaus Lucke Horst Laqua

# Silicone Oil in the Treatment of Complicated Retinal Detachments

## Techniques, Results, and Complications

With 44 Figures (12 in color), and 15 Tables

Springer-Verlag Berlin Heidelberg New York
London Paris Tokyo Hong Kong Barcelona

Priv. Doz. Dr. med. Klaus Lucke, M.B. Ch.B.
Professor Dr. med. Horst Laqua

Klinik für Augenheilkunde
der Medizinischen Universität zu Lübeck
Ratzeburger Allee 160
D-2400 Lübeck 1

ISBN 3-540-53035-5 Springer-Verlag Berlin Heidelberg New York
ISBN 0-387-53035-5 Springer-Verlag New York Berlin Heidelberg



2125/3145-543210 - Printed on acid-free paper

# Foreword

Silicone oil was introduced into ophthalmic surgery by Paul Cibis in the early 1960's in an attempt to treat giant retinal tears and cases where retinal detachment had failed to respond to conventional scleral buckling techniques. His understanding of the nature of vitreous pathology and how it related to complex retinal detachment laid the foundation for modern vitreoretinal surgery.

Cibis's success with these problems together with his rationale for separating membranes from the retina led others to try their hand at learning his techniques. At the same time much criticism was levelled at the concept of injecting what was regarded as a foreign material into the eye, as well as to the whole idea of operating within the vitreous cavity. Some of this was personal, some due to a lack of understanding of the underlying pathology and some due to disappointment following surgical failure using the new methods.

Early results were certainly encouraging but it was not until the advent of pars plana vitrectomy that it became possible to develop more refined methods in combination with the use silicone oil so that much better results could be obtained.

The introduction of pars plana vitrectomy where instruments were used to peel membranes had been hoped to achieve as good, if not better results than with silicone oil, but proved not be the case. After membrane peeling gas was used to provide a temporary retinal tamponade in the hope of stabilising the reattached retina. However recurrences were common, and surgeons began to look again at the need for a more permanent material as a substitute for gas.

The case against silicone was re-examined and animal work repeated, this time using operated controls, and the main concern that silicone was toxic to the retina was abandoned. Thus silicone oil became respectable and is now widely used by retinal surgeons involved in the treatment of complex cases.

Klaus Lucke and Horst Laqua are two such doctors who have been working for some years in this area. Their book is the culmination of this work and provides an excellent exposition of the current state of the art in vitreoretinal surgery using silicone oil.

Their analysis is based on very nearly five hundred patients with a wide variety of pathology, ranging from proliferative vitreoretinopathy through giant breaks to the late complications of diabetic retinopathy; the rationale and technique for each is considered in detail, and there are excellent line diagrams to illustrate all important points. Some unusual cases are included which extend the use of silicone oil beyond what may now be regarded as the conventional.

Results are described in great detail, and the very important aspect of the need in some cases for more than one operation to achieve a stable result is rightly emphasised. Their results are very good indeed and are compared and contrasted with those of other workers.

Complications are analysed in detail and confirm earlier observations that many problems which commonly follow the use of silicone are due to pathological changes resulting from the underlying disease. Others are avoidable by the use of more careful technique. Only a few problems, such as emulsification, are directly attributable to the silicone material itself.

The discussion section is a comprehensive review of every possible aspect of the use of silicone oil. The literature is totally reviewed and discussed. No complication or criticism is ignored, and no ophthalmologist who has any concern regarding the place of silicone oil in the surgery of complex retinal detachment could be left in any doubt that Dr. Lucke and Dr. Laqua have carefully considered all aspects of its use before recommending it in these complex and desperate cases.

The problem of silicone oil removal is discussed in a very practical manner, highlighting the difficulty which many patients have in accepting the current recommendation that silicone oil should be removed in all cases. Many cannot accept the significant risk of recurrence of a problem which only silicone oil has been able to successfully treat, perhaps after several conventional operations on an only eye.

Perhaps the most telling section of the book is the shortest, and is to be found in the last paragraph; this refers to future improvements and the need for better primary care of retinal detachment and of diabetic retinopathy. The need for complex vitreoretinal surgery could largely be prevented by improved primary care. Most PVR is due to failed conventional surgery where breaks have not been identified or treated using inadequate or inappropriate primary surgical technique. Most late complications of diabetic retinopathy could be prevented by laser therapy carried out in an appropriate manner at the correct time. It is in the field of prevention that future development should lie.

For the present however there is a continuing need for silicone oil combined with vitrectomy instrumentation and Klaus Lucke and Horst Laqua are to be congratulated on a superbly presented book which provides a major contribution to our ophthalmic literature.

John D. Scott, FRCS
Consultant Ophthalmic Surgeon.
Addenbrooks Hospital, Cambridge.

# Contents

# Color Plates

## Color Plate 1

**Fig. 1a.** *Proliferative vitreoretinopathy* stage D3, funnel shaped retinal detachment with full thickness folds in all four quadrants and partially pigmented preretinal membranes; preoperative view of the fundus

**Fig. 1b.** The same eye 1 year after initial surgery: encircling band, pars plana vitrectomy, membrane peeling, silicone oil filling; removal of silicone oil after 1 year; retinal reattachment, visual acuity 0.2

**Fig. 2a.** *Giant tear*, preoperative view of the fundus; retina is folded over. Upper half; free view of the underlying pigment epithelium, lower half; view of the reverse side of the retina

**Fig 2b.** The same eye 1 month after surgery: encircling band, pars plana vitrectomy, silicone oil filling; retinal reattachment, visual acuity 0.1

**Fig. 3a.** *Posterior hole*, preoperative view of the fundus; radial tear can be seen nasal to the optic disc in an area of chorioretinal atrophy; previous surgery with vitrectomy and gas failed

**Fig. 3b.** The same eye 3 weeks after surgery: silicone oil filling with endodiathermy to the retinal edge and underlying choroid; retinal reattachment. visual acuity 1/20

# Color Plate 1

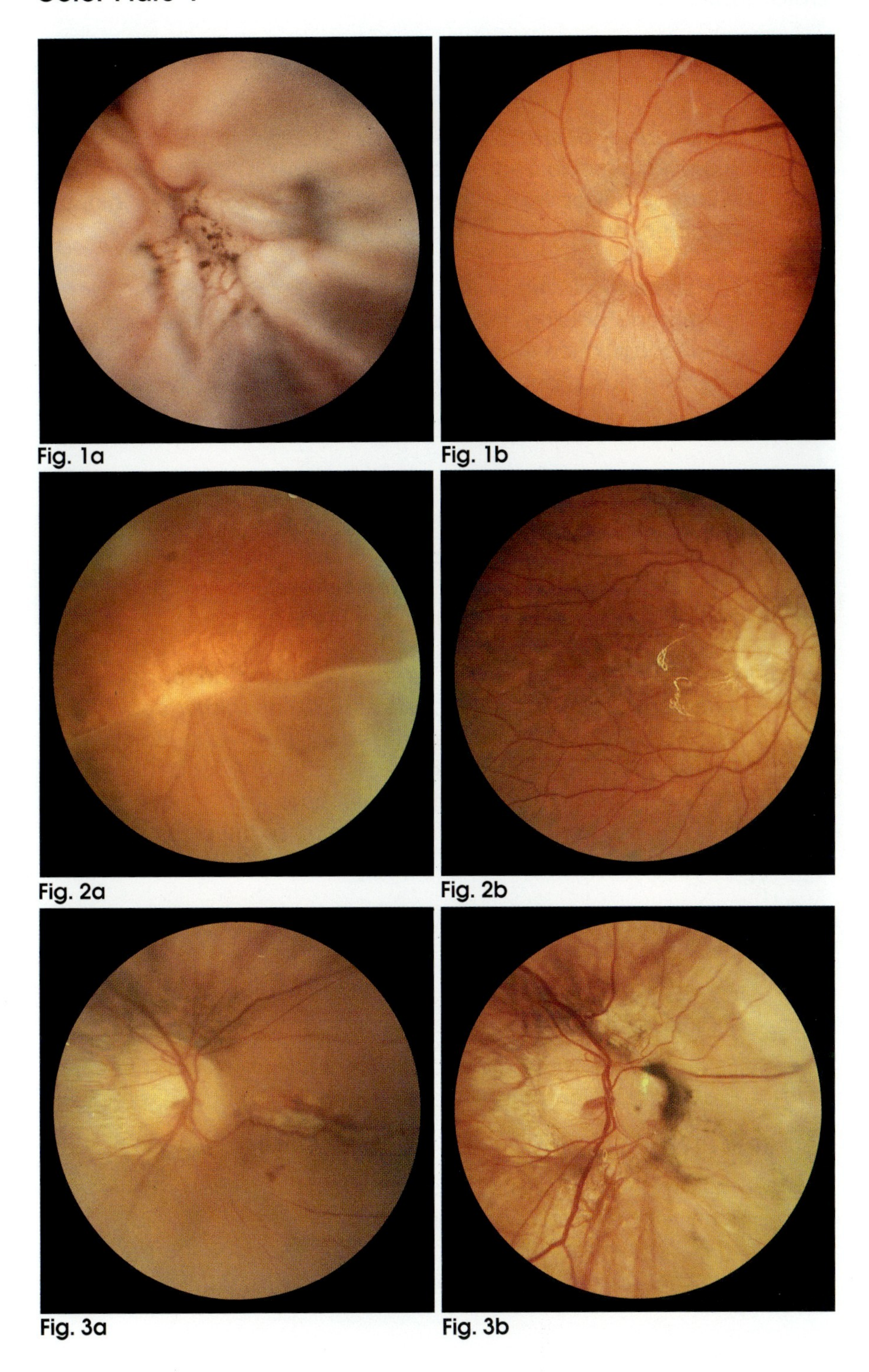

Fig. 1a

Fig. 1b

Fig. 2a

Fig. 2b

Fig. 3a

Fig. 3b

## Color Plate 2

**Fig. 1a.** *Proliferative diabetic retinopathy*, young female patient with massively vascularized preretinal proliferations at high risk of developing postoperative hemorrhage and neovascular glaucoma; preoperative view of the fundus

**Fig. 1b.** The same eye 3 years after initial surgery: pars plana vitrectomy, membrane peeling, silicone oil filling, postoperative panretinal laser coagulation; removal of silicone oil and cataract 1 year later; retinal reattachment, optic atrophy, visual acuity 0.2

**Fig. 2a.** *Proliferative diabetic retinopathy*, patient with particularly dense preretinal membranes, thin, atrophic retina underneath and traction detachment; preoperative view of the fundus

**Fig 2b.** The same eye 3 days after surgery: encircling band, pars plana vitrectomy, silicone oil filling, retinectomy, endolaser coagulation to retinectomy edge; retinal reattachment, visual acuity 1/50. The retina has remained attached subsequently and the retinectomy edge scarred over without complications; the silicone oil and the lens were removed 15 months later; the visual acuity stabilized at 0.1

**Fig. 3a.** *Perforating injury*, redetachment with PVR after surgery with vitrectomy and gas, note massive retinal contraction and membrane proliferation along the edge of the encircling buckle; preoperative view of the fundus;

**Fig. 3b.** The same eye 1 week after surgery: large circumferential retinectomy with removal of contracted peripheral retina to relieve antero-posterior traction, silicone oil filling, endodiathermy to the retinal edge; retinal reattachment, visual acuity 0.1

## Color Plate 2

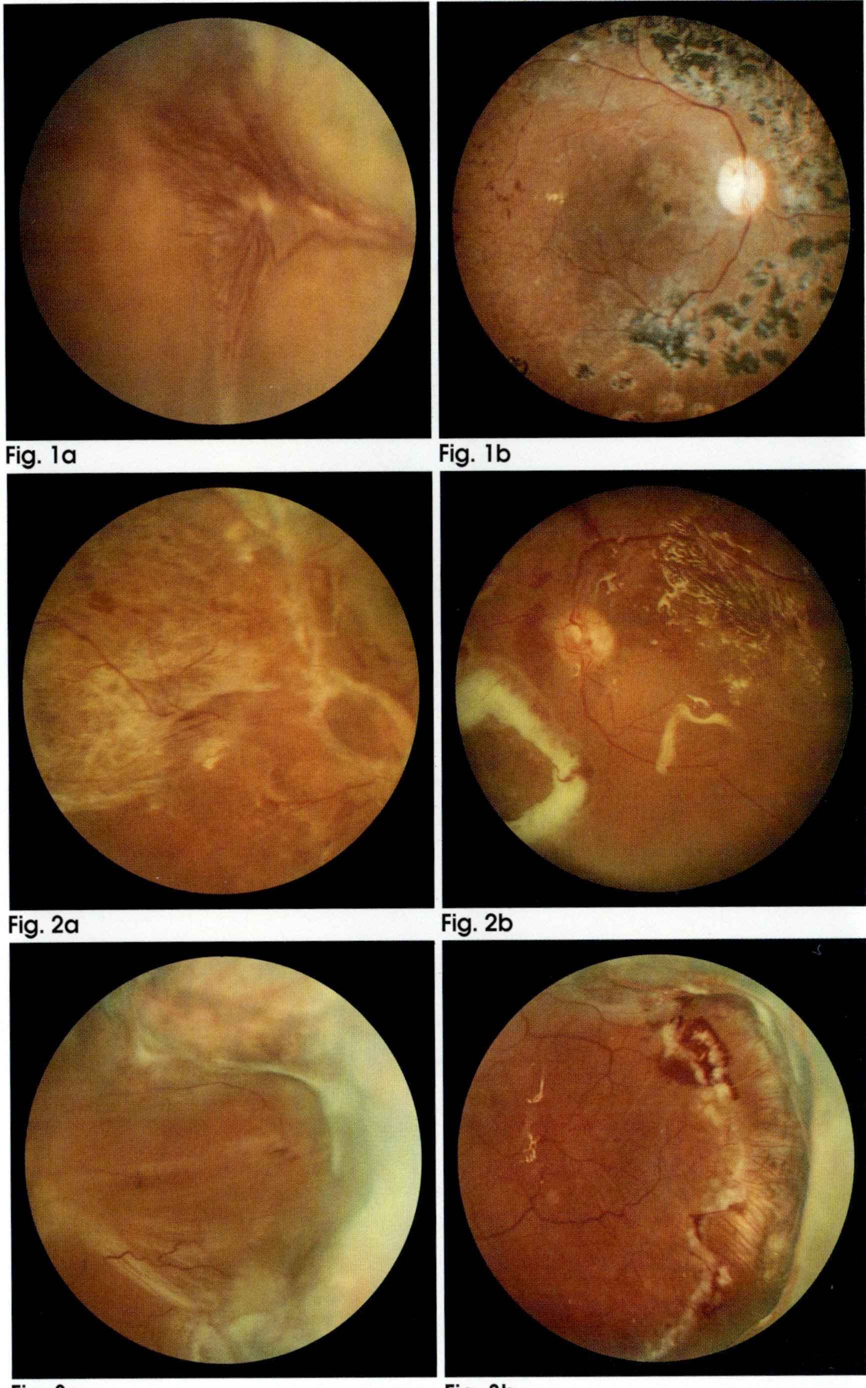

Fig. 1a

Fig. 1b

Fig. 2a

Fig. 2b

Fig. 3a

Fig. 3b

## Color Plate 3

**Fig. 1a.** *Adequate silicone oil filling:* postoperative view of an eye filled adequately with silicone oil, note silicone oil reflex at the edge of the encircling buckle

**Fig. 1b.** *Inadequate silicone oil filling:* postoperative view of an eye filled inadequately with silicone oil, note large space between silicone oil bubble and encircling buckle; high risk of reproliferation and redetachment

**Fig. 2a.** *Reproliferation in an eye with PVR filled with silicone oil:* note typically flat, white, densely packed membranes

**Fig 2b.** *Histology of preretinal membrane* taken from an enucleated eye with silicone oil and redetached retina: note round, empty spaces probably representing silicone oil vacuoles in the preretinal membrane overlying disorganized gliotic retina showing no evidence of intraretinal silicone oil

**Fig. 3a.** *Segmental cataract in an eye filled with silicone oil:* note opacification of the lens in the left upper quadrant, in the area where silicone oil is in contact with the lens.

**Fig. 3b.** View of the fundus of the same eye: note small silicone oil bubble in the upper half of the vitreous space. The eye was operated on 20 years ago with the original Cibis technique; visual acuity 0.2

## Color Plate 3

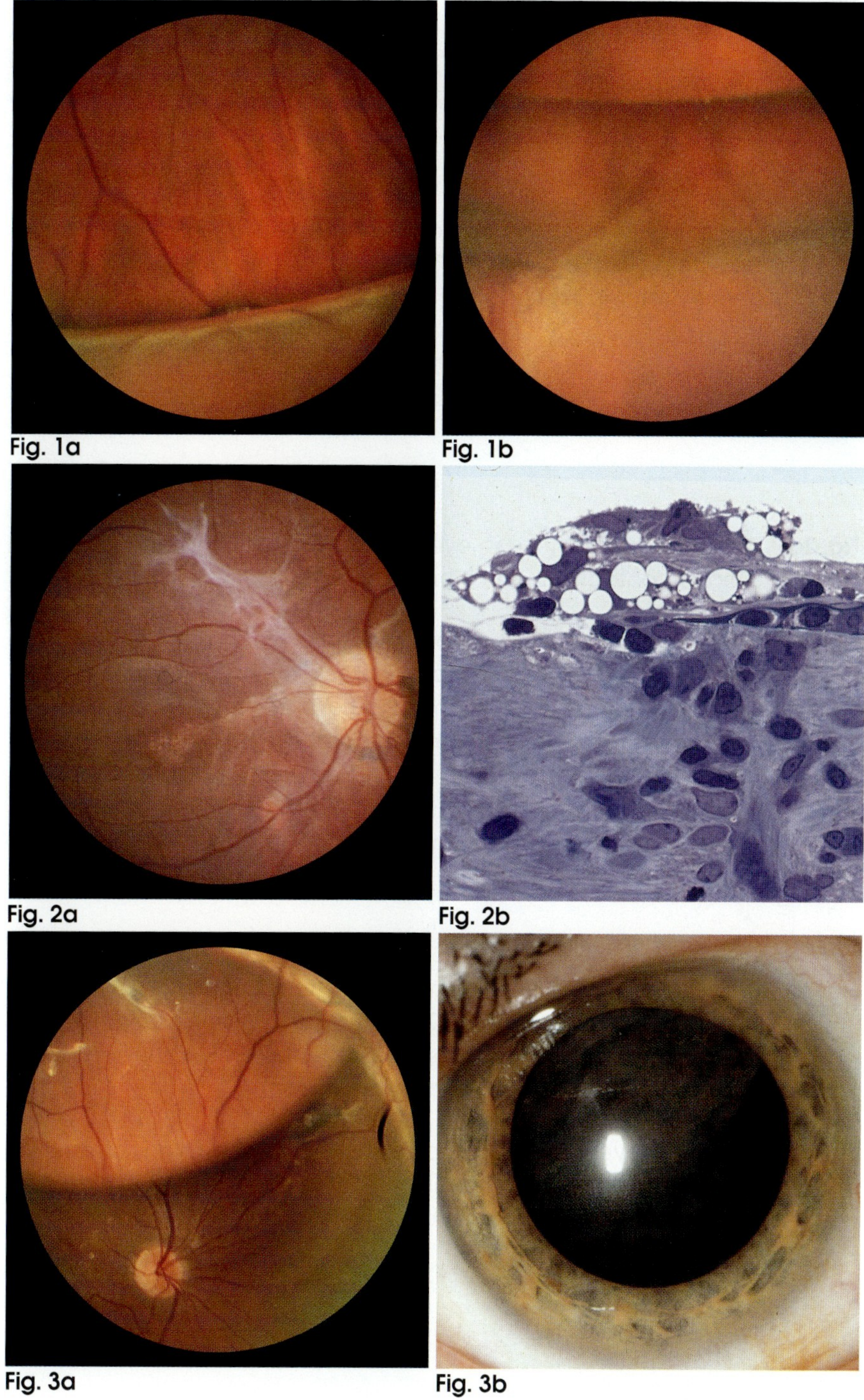

Fig. 1a
Fig. 1b
Fig. 2a
Fig. 2b
Fig. 3a
Fig. 3b

## Color Plate 4

**Fig. 1a.** *Silicone oil prolapse into the anterior chamber* in an aphakic eye filled with silicone oil and spontaneously occluded Ando iridectomy

**Fig. 1a.** The same eye 20 minutes after reopening of the inferior basal iridectomy with a pulsed Nd:YAG laser, the silicone oil has spontaneously returned behind the pupillary plane

**Fig. 2a.** *Band keratopathy* in an eye with silicone oil filling and long-term silicone contact with the corneal endothelium

**Fig 2b.** *Bullous keratopathy* due to endothelial decompensation in the same eye 24 hours after silicone oil removal. The endothelial decompensation had been masked by silicone oil filling the entire anterior chamber and preventing corneal hydration

**Fig. 3a.** *Emulsification* with "inverse hypopion" formation in an eye operated on with *silicone oil OP1000* for RDP and combined traction and rhegmatogenous detachment 12 months previously (retina has redetached due to massive reproliferation)

**Fig. 3b.** The other eye of the same patient without overt signs of emulsification. This eye had undergone the same procedure for the same situation with *silicone oil OP5000* 15 months previously (here also now redetachment)

## Color Plate 4

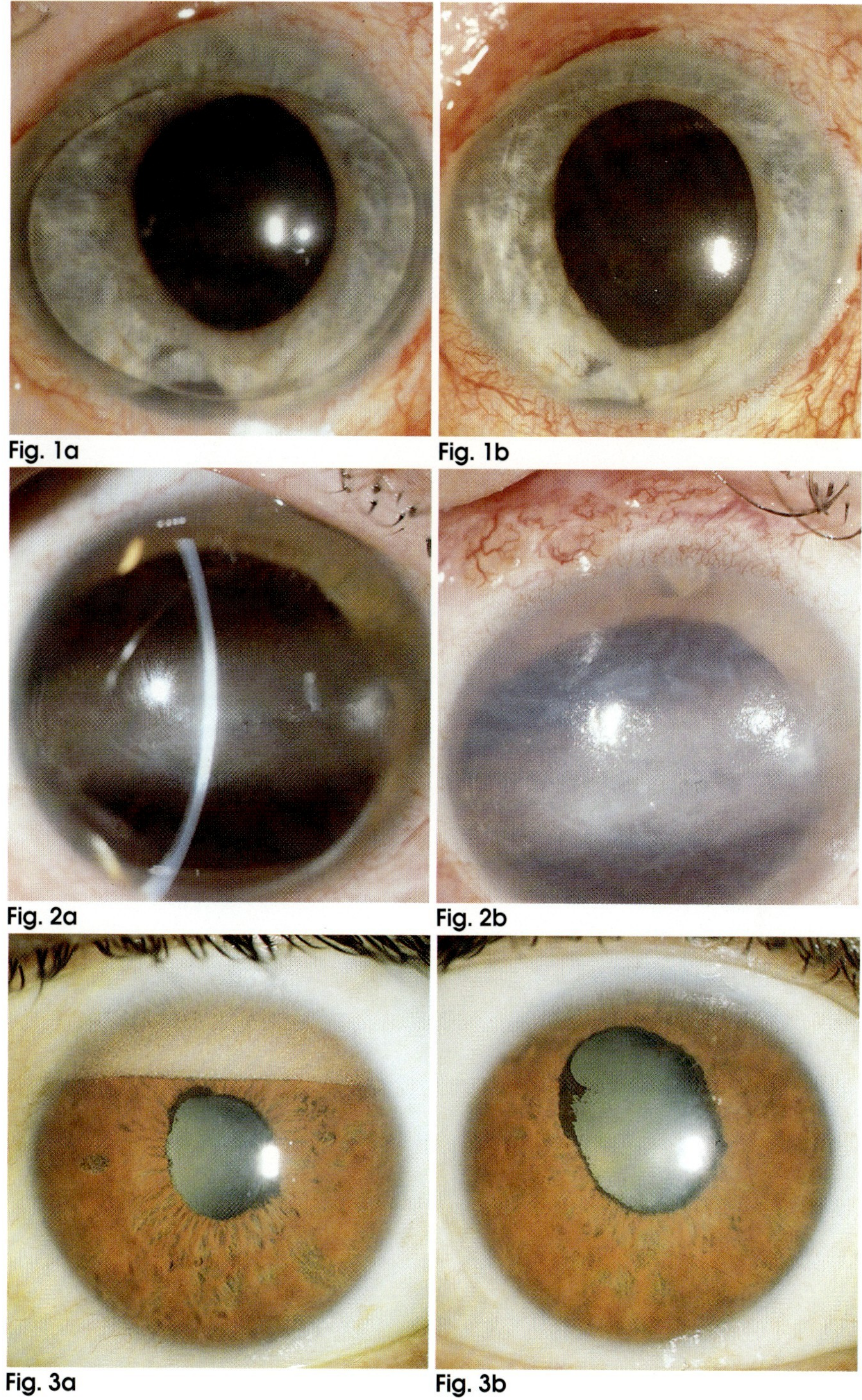

Fig. 1a

Fig. 1b

Fig. 2a

Fig. 2b

Fig. 3a

Fig. 3b

# 1 Introduction

The history of the surgical treatment of retinal detachments can from today's point of view be divided into three phases. In the first phase, lasting from about 1923 to 1970, the principles of what is known as *conventional retinal surgery* were developed. By these primarily extraocular measures the retina could be reattached, somewhat indirectly, with a good rate of success in uncomplicated cases. In the second phase, lasting from about 1970 to 1980, vitreous surgery was developed. It was thus possible for the first time to treat retinal detachments from within the eye to remove opacities or membranes or to manipulate the retina directly, thereby treating surgically what up to then had been considered inoperable. The third phase commenced around the beginning of the 1980s and seems to have now reached an end point. It is characterized by the introduction of direct retinal surgery and internal long-term tamponade with gas or silicone oil. By this so-called extreme vitreoretinal surgery, successful treatment of the remaining complicated retinal detachments may be possible.

## 1.1 Conventional Retinal Surgery

The basic principles of retinal surgery, still valid today, were formulated by Gonin (1923) and consist of closure of the retinal tear, drainage of subretinal fluid, and coagulation to seal the edges of the tear permanently. After exact localization of the tear, Gonin incised the sclera, drained the subretinal fluid through a sclerotomy, and then used hot diathermy to coagulate the retina directly. With this method he was able to cure 40% of his patients – a sensation in those days.

Further development was aimed at optimizing closure of the tear and fixation of the retina. Rosengren's method (1938) of attaching the retina by means of intraocularly injected air and tamponading retinal holes with air from the inside did not get much response in those days and has only been taken up again in more recent times (Hilton and Grizzard 1986). Galezowski's idea (1890) of sewing the retina to the sclera was also too progressive for his time and was only tried again very much later in the context of extreme vitreoretinal surgery (Usui et al. 1977, Federman et al. 1982).

Buckling retinal surgery, introduced by Custodis in 1953, determined the course of further development. By sewing an explant onto the sclera, the tear, pretreated by diathermy, was closed and, at the same time, vitreous traction was relieved. By this method Custodis achieved a success rate of 84% in selected eyes.

Further technical improvements were the introduction of binocular indirect ophthalmoscopy (Schepens 1947), the introduction of encircling bands at the end of the 1950s (Schepens 1964), improved buckling material made of elastic silicone sponge (Lincoff et al. 1965), and, most of all, the substitution of the very destructive diathermy treatment with light coagulation (Meyer-Schwickerath 1959) and cryocoagulation (Lincoff et al. 1964).

Thus, so-called conventional retinal surgery has developed into a standard procedure consisting of buckling (encircling band/sponge explants), drainage of the subretinal fluid, and coagulation of the retinal tear edges (cryo-, light, or laser coagulation).

Since the end of the 1960s, methods have been available which are still routinely applied and by which 80%-90% of all primary retinal detachments can be cured.

## 1.2 Vitreous Surgery

These therapeutic measures were, however, not sufficient for the remaining 10% to 20% of detachments. Fundamentally new treatment modalities were needed to deal surgically with eyes that had one or a combination of the following complicating factors:

1. Optical problems, e.g., opacity (cataract) or vitreous hemorrhage, obstructing the view to the retina and thus preventing a planned buckling procedure
2. Traction membranes on or under the retina, e.g., proliferative vitreoretinopathy or proliferative diabetic retinopathy, which mechanically prevent reattachment of the retina
3. Large retinal holes, e.g., giant tears of 90° or more, which cannot be satisfactorily tamponaded with a circumferential buckle
4. Posteriorly located holes which cannot be buckled satisfactorily due to their location at the posterior pole

The first practical surgical concept for these complications was developed by Kasner, who with simple instruments removed the vitreous subtotally through the pupil after having removed the cornea and the lens. His report on the first two eyes treated by this so-called open-sky vitrectomy (Kasner et al. 1968) was, from today's point of view, a historical step. Not only did it demonstrate that the eye could tolerate such a procedure and the removal of the vitreous body, but also that the surgical method was in considerable need of improvement. This development then led to modern vitreous surgery, which was influenced to a large extent by Machemer and his colleagues (1971); however, others (e.g., Klöti, Peyman, Charles and Schepens and their colleagues) also made important contributions.

Today, the technique of vitreous surgery has been perfected to quite an extent, and with special tools and instruments lens and vitreous can be removed by small incisions in the pars plana, membranes can be peeled from the retina, and the retina itself can be touched, manipulated, or even cut (Machemer and Aaberg 1981, Michels 1981, Schepens 1983, Charles 1981).

Since the end of the 1970s this development has come technically and conceptionally to a conclusion, and the complications mentioned above can be cured 60% – 80% of the time by vitreous surgical techniques.

## 1.3 Extreme Vitreoretinal Surgery

It soon became evident, however, that although many complicated retinal detachments could now be treated much better surgically, the anatomic long-term results were often disappointing (Machemer 1977, Ratner et al. 1983). The problems were, to some extent, technical problems at the time of surgery, but persistent reproliferation leading to renewed membrane growth and redetachment of the retina occurred after weeks or months and limited the rate of success.

Thus, at the end of the 1970s an end point had again been reached at which it became evident that the remaining patients and those being added because of ever expanding indications (proliferative vitreoretinopathy, giant tears, posterior holes, proliferative diabetic retinopathy, perforating injuries), could not be operated on with sufficient chance of lasting success by pure vitrectomy techniques alone.

Since then development has continued on different tracks. For example it has been attempted to *check reproliferation medically or by radia-*

*tion*. Numerous cytotoxic agents, corticosteroids, and antiphlogistics have been tested, using animal models, as to their effectiveness in attenuating proliferation. Only a few substances were effective enough and of low enough toxicity that clinical trials could be considered. Thus, oral colchicine (Lemor et al. 1987), 5-fluorouracil (Blumenkranz et al. 1984, Tavakolian and Wollensak 1985), oral prednisolone (Körner et al. 1982), intraocular triamcinolone (Tano et al. 1980, Chandler et al. 1987), and daunomycin (Kirmani et al. 1983) have been tested as to their suitability. In this context the first clinical experiments by Wiedemann, Heimann, and colleagues at the Cologne Ophthalmologic Clinic (1987a, b) with daunomycin are promising. Experiments treating proliferative vitreoretinopathy with high energy radiation are still in the early stages and have so far only been effective to a limited extent (Binder et al. 1988b). Furthermore it became evident that both additional *aggressive surgical techniques and intraocular long-term tamponade* were necessary to improve the long-term surgical success rates.

Repeated attempts have been made, some a long time ago, to replace pathologically altered vitreous by other substances, hoping thereby to relieve traction or to tamponade retinal defects from within. Thus, Ohm tried to inject air into the vitreous cavity as early as 1911; others tried injections of sodium chloride (Grossman 1883, Birch-Hirschfeld 1912), animal vitreous (Deutschmann 1906), cerebrospinal fluid (Fritz 1947), human vitreous (Paufique 1953, Shafer 1957, and Cutler 1946), polyvinylpyrolidone (Hayano and Voschino 1959), hyaluronic acid (Widder 1960 and Hruby 1961), and polyacrylamide (Müller-Jensen 1968).

All these substances had, however, been injected into the eye without prior removal of the vitreous body. Some were unable to fulfil a tamponading function because they lacked surface tension towards water (e.g. sodium chloride, cerebrospinal fluid, and hyaluronic acid), were absorbed too quickly (air), or were too toxic (polyvinylpyrolidone, polyacrylamide). Only silicone oil or gases of long duration have been used successfully to date as substances suitable for long-term tamponade in vitrectomized eyes.

### 1.3.1 Silicone Oil in Retinal Surgery

Cibis, taking up the idea of vitreous substitution, had already in the early 1960s injected silicone oil into eyes with proliferative vitreoretinopathy. On the basis of experiments by Poleman and Froitzheim (1953), who proved that silicone oil was biologically well-tolerated, and the experiments by Stone (1962) and Armaly (1962a, b), who demonstrated good intraocular tolerance to silicone oil, he injected silicone oil with a syringe into the space between the preretinal membranes and the retina under indirect binocular ophthalmoscopic observation (Cibis et al. 1962, Cibis 1964, 1965). In this way, the hydraulic power of the oil was used to peel the membranes off the retina and to press the retina onto the underlying pigment epithelium (virtually a vitreous procedure), at the same time using the oil to tamponade existing retinal holes permanently. The necessary volume was gained by simultaneously draining the subretinal fluid externally through the sclera. With this method, surprising success was achieved in eyes which were considered inoperable in those days. For the first time it was possible to treat "massive vitreous retraction" (proliferative vitreoretinopathy) and giant tears.

Cibis' method was taken up by many and caused a sensation (Levine and Ellis 1963, Bonnet 1964, Höpping 1964, Moreau 1964, Lund 1968, Liesenhoff 1968, Meyer-Schwickerath et al. 1969, Cockerham et al. 1969, Kanski and Daniel 1973). It proved, however, to be technically extremely difficult and was certainly not performed by all emulators with comparable skill. Reports of serious complications with silicone oil in plastic surgery of the breast, in which implantations of silicone prostheses led to severe tissue reactions with macrophage and giant cell formation (Wilflingseder et al. 1974, Wintsch et al. 1978), soon resulted in a prohibition of silicone oil by the Food and Drug Administration. Disappointing functional results, high rates of complications (Watzke 1967a, Okun 1968, Cockerham et al. 1969, Kanski and Daniel 1973, Sugar and Okamura 1976), reports on intraretinal silicone oil (Lee et al. 1969, Blodi 1971, Mukai et al. 1972), and Cibis' early death all contributed to the method being discontinued in the USA after only a few years.

In Europe, some patients had also been operated on with silicone oil in the sixties and, there also, the method proved too difficult, especially since in Europe binocular indirect ophthalmoscopy was not used at the time. Accordingly, the results were disappointing, rates of complications high, and histologic examinations of operated on eyes showed alarming permeations of all tissues with silicone droplets (Lund 1968, Rentsch et.al 1977, Manschot 1978, Alexandridis and Daniel 1981).

John Scott in Cambridge was the only one to continue and develop Cibis' method in the 1970s (Scott 1977). He used the binocular indirect ophthalmoscope and also designed a number of instruments (e.g., microscissors) with which he could perform intraocular manipulations. He too injected the oil with a syringe under binocular ophthalmoscopy in eyes that had not been vitrectomized. The silicone oil was left in the eye permanently. The widespread use of his method was, however, prevented by the high expectations the newly developed vitreous surgery elicited in the USA and by publications on late complications in eyes having been operated on with silicone oil in the 1960s.

The credit for combining vitreous surgery and silicone oil tamponade into a new concept for the therapy of complicated retinal detachments goes largely to Relja Živojnović in Rotterdam (Živojnović et al. 1981+1982), who called it a "logical consequence" (1987). Decisive was the realization that relief of retinal traction and manipulation of the retina were not possible without vitreous surgery and that the subsequent silicone oil tamponade made the development of increasingly courageous maneuvers possible, including cutting the retina or even removing part of it – up to then an unimaginable surgical step. This combination of direct retinal surgery and long-term tamponade is referred to today as extreme vitreoretinal surgery.

Since the early 1980s many European vitreoretinal surgeons, who were convinced by the work of Živojnović, have cooperated closely and advanced silicone oil surgery against prevailing American opinion. Besides Relja Živojnović in Rotterdam they are: John Scott (Cambridge), Peter Leaver (London), Klaus Heimann (Cologne), Philipp Sourdille (Nantes), Michel Gonvers (Lausanne), Philipp Cleary (Dublin), Jürgen Faulborn (Basel), and our group (Essen/Lübeck). Others have since joined.

## 1.3.2 Long-Acting Gases in Vitreoretinal Surgery

As a result of negative publicity and the early prohibition of silicone oil in the USA by the FDA, the development there took a different turn and attempts were made to achieve long-term tamponade using gases of long intraocular duration. At the end of the 1970s it had already been attempted to improve the results with an intraocular tamponade of air or sulfur hexafluoride gas ($SF_6$) in vitrectomized eyes (Fineberg et al. 1975, Machemer and Laqua 1978, Abrams et al. 1982). The half-lives of intraocular air and $SF_6$ bubbles at 2 and 4 days, respectively, are too short, however, so that gases were needed that would remain in the eye longer. A number of perfluorocarbons were tested as to their suitability: octafluorocyclobutane, $C_4F_8$ (Peyman et al. 1975a); perfluoromethane, $CF_4$ (H. Lincoff et al. 1983); perfluoroethane, $C_2F_6$ (H. Lincoff et. al. 1983); perfluoropropane, $C_3F_8$ (H. Lincoff et. al. 1983, Chang et al. 1984, Faulborn and Bowald 1987); and perfluoro-n-butane, $C_4F_{10}$ (H. Lincoff et. al. 1983). All of these gases are chemically inert and expand in pure form in the eye. With suitable mixtures stable intraocular gas bubbles of different half-lives can be obtained. For clinical use $C_2F_6$ (half-life 6 days), $C_3F_8$ (half-life 10 days), and $C_4F_{10}$ (half- life 20 days) have been generally accepted in the USA and are used in certain situations by us as well. The main advantage of long-acting gases is the fact that they resorb spontaneously and need not be removed from the eye by an additional operation. But just this is also their major disadvantage: a stable, controlled, long-term tamponade cannot be achieved. Strangely enough the above-mentioned gases have also not yet been approved by the FDA for intraocular application.

The controversy between American and European vitreous surgeons concerning the respective advantages and disadvantages of intraocular gas and silicone oil tamponade has not been entirely settled to date. Lately, however, there has been a certain degree of reconciliation because, firstly, silicone oil is usually removed after several months while gases are spontaneously resorbed; secondly, there is a growing trend towards the use of silicone oil for certain indications even in the USA; and thirdly, silicone oil surgery has also become an accepted form of therapy today in the USA, its development being complete and thus no longer considered as an experimental method.

# 2 Materials and Methods

## 2.1 Silicone Oils

### 2.1.1 Properties of Silicone Oils

#### 2.1.1.1 Chemistry

All silicone oils used clinically in recent years are composed of the same basic molecule: polydimethylsiloxane (PDMS). It is transparent with a refractive index of 1.404 and is somewhat lighter than water (specific gravity = 0.97). It is permeable to oxygen and has a high surface tension towards air (21 mN/m) and water (40 mN/m) and, accordingly, does not mix with them. In pure form it largely exhibits those properties an ophthalmologic implant material should ideally posses: chemically largely inert, completely permeable to light in the visible light spectrum, biologically not degradable in tissue, not carcinogenic, mechanically stable, and easily sterilizable due to its high heat resistance (Habal et al. 1980, Kreiner 1987). Other silicone oils, e.g., fluoro- or phenylsilicones, are still in the experimental stage and have properties that make clinical application at present inadvisable (Petersen et al. 1986, Gabel et al. 1987b).

PDMS is a polymer of dimethylsiloxane subunits. Through polymerization of dimethylsiloxane units it becomes polydimethylsiloxane:

$$HO-\underset{CH_3}{\overset{CH_3}{Si}}-\boxed{OH + H}O-\underset{CH_3}{\overset{CH_3}{Si}}-OH + \ldots \xrightarrow[-H_2O]{} -O-\underset{CH_3}{\overset{CH_3}{Si}}-O-\underset{CH_3}{\overset{CH_3}{Si}}-O\left[\underset{CH_3}{\overset{CH_3}{Si}}-O\right]_x$$

It is then completed by interrupting the polymerization process with end-blocking trimethylsiloxane units:

$$\begin{array}{c} CH_3 \\ | \\ -Si- \\ | \\ CH_3 \end{array} O \begin{array}{c} CH_3 \\ | \\ -Si- \\ | \\ CH_3 \end{array} \boxed{OH + H} O \begin{array}{c} CH_3 \\ | \\ -Si- \\ | \\ CH_3 \end{array} CH_3 \xrightarrow[-H_2O]{} \left[ \begin{array}{c} CH_3 \\ | \\ Si \\ | \\ CH_3 \end{array} - O \right] \begin{array}{c} CH_3 \\ | \\ Si \\ | \\ CH_3 \end{array} - O - \begin{array}{c} CH_3 \\ | \\ Si \\ | \\ CH_3 \end{array} - CH_3$$

The lengths of the chains depend on the duration of the polymerization process, which thus affects the viscosity of the material as well. PDMS with lower molecular weight is liquid, while substances with higher molecular weight are viscous to highly viscous. Cross-linked PDMS chains are rubber-like materials (silicone rubber). They are, for instance, used to produce encircling bands and lately are also implanted as flexible intraocular lenses.

While it is possible to achieve a certain desired viscosity with a certain molecular chain length, the same viscosity can be acquired by mixing two different silicone oils of higher and lower viscosity (Kreiner 1987). This leads to the important conclusion that two silicone oils of different production batches will not have the same composition even though they might have identical viscosities. The statistical distribution of molecular chain lengths in a silicone oil charge can be determined by gel chromatographic separation (Fig. 1). A simpler process to obtain an indication of the composition of a silicone oil is to determine its volatility. The higher the proportion of short molecular chains in an oil, the higher will be the loss of mass if the oil is heated to 200°C for 24 h (Gabel et al. 1987a).

The biological tolerance of a silicone oil depends on a variety of factors. First, the proportion of short molecular chains in the oil is important. Whereas high molecular weight PDMS evidently possesses an excellent tissue tolerance, short molecular chains may emulsify (Crisp et al. 1987) or diffuse into the tissue and cause reactions there. Second, the purity of the material is important. Unpolymerized monomeric dimethylsiloxanes, cyclic low molecular weight siloxanes, a high proportion of chemically very reactive OH groups, and catalytic remnants, primarily heavy metal ions, all are characterized by a high toxic potential (Kreiner 1987). Production should therefore attach considerable importance to complete polymerization, full removal of catalytic components, and a low proportion of low molecular weight and cyclic siloxanes.

Measurements of the electrical resistance, which are dependent on the concentration of heavy metal ions, serve as another indicator of the purity of the material. The higher the resistance, the fewer catalytic remnants in the sample (Gabel et al. 1987a).

It is regrettable that a great number of different silicone oils have been used since the first operation by Cibis in 1962 (Gabel et al. 1987a). In some cases the origin of particular oils can no longer be traced nor can their purity and composition be measured. In Europe we and most of the other surgeons have used the silicone oil General Electric SF 96 since 1979. In 1980 the Wacker company, in cooperation with the Munich Ophthalmologic Clinic, developed two oils (viscosity 1000 and 5000 cps, respectively) from which, in a special process, the short molecular chains (molecular weight of less than 2400) were largely removed ("purified", Fig. 1). At first those oils were only used in Munich; however, since 1984 we have also employed the purified OP5000 which, beginning in 1986 has been produced in an improved form by the Adatomed company in Munich. In this oil the amount of free OH endgroups has been reduced to a minimum and standardized. Furthermore, by an improved purification and sterilization process, an oil free of pyrogen and constant with regard to the distribution of chain lengths has been developed, in which decomposition during sterilization has been eliminated.

A study by Gabel and colleagues (1987a), examining 14 silicone oils of different origins, showed that the grades of purity of silicone oils used by various surgeons worldwide differed significantly. The proportion of short molecular chains ranged between 3.4% (a Belgian oil), 1.5% (General Electric SF96), and 0% (Wacker OP1000, OP5000). Volatility amounted to 1.6% for SF96 and <0.05% for the Wacker oils; and electric resistance was $2 \times 10^{14}\ \Omega$ for SF96 and $3 \times 10^{15}\ \Omega$ for the Wacker oils (Table 1).

These highly differing grades of purity may explain the different experiences encountered by various surgeons and some of the contradictory results of experimental studies. Especially with regard to postoperative complications, e.g., emulsification, secondary glaucoma, and keratopathy, these differences could very well be relevant. At the moment the two purified oils (OP1000 and OP5000) possess the best properties among the oils available, as far as they are measurable, and, accordingly, should be used exclusively. As more highly viscous oils show a considerably lower tendency to emulsify (Crisp et al. 1987), since October 1984 we have used only OP5000, and, since March 1987 its additionally improved form (see Color Plate 4, Figs. 3a + b).

**Table 1.** Properties of clinically used silicone oils

| | |
|---|---|
| Refractive index | 1.404 |
| Specific weight | 0.97 |
| Surface tension | 21 mN/m towards air<br>40 mN/m towards water |
| Volatility(200°C/24 h) | <0.05% – 1.6% |
| Volume resistance(23°C) | $2 \times 10^{14}\ \Omega - 3 \times 10^{15}\ \Omega$ |
| Short molecular chains (MW<2400) | 0% – 3.4% |

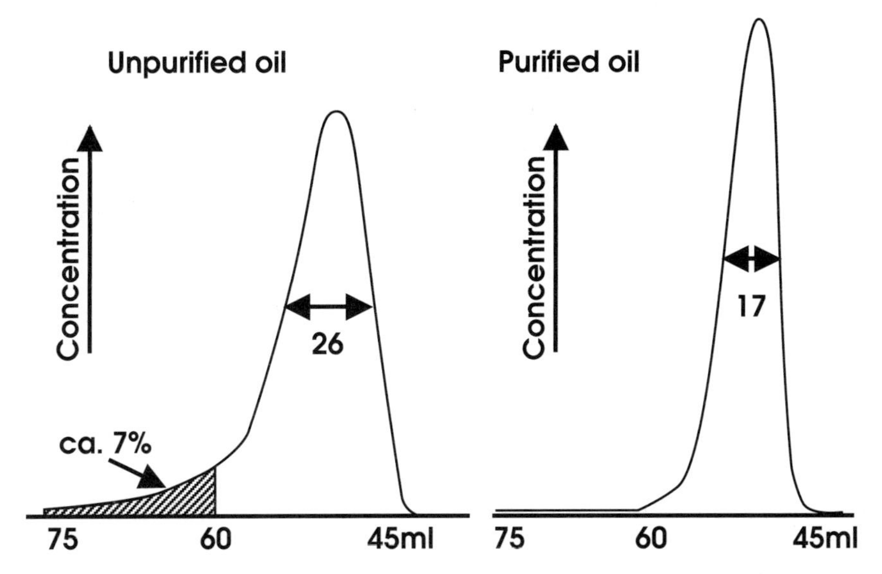


**Fig. 1.** GPC (gel permeation chromatogram) of an unpurified and a purified silicone oil. The unpurified oil contains about 7% low molecular weight chains which have been almost totally removed from the purified oil. Furthermore, the peak of the curve of the purified oil is narrower (half-width = 17) indicating greater homogeneity of the chain lengths (from Kreiner 1987)

### 2.1.1.2 Optics

As the refractive index of silicone oil (1.404) is higher than that of vitreous and aqueous humor, the optics of an eye will change when filled with silicone. The calculations are very complex and cannot be made accurately even if performed with great care since the curvature of the anterior silicone oil surface cannot be measured and, moreover, it can change, especially in the aphakic eye, depending on posture. As a general rule, in the phakic eye the concave front surface of the silicone oil in contact with the lens causes a hyperopic change in refraction (to about +5 diopters), whereas an aphakic eye becomes myopic by the now convex silicone oil front surface (to about +5 diopters residual refraction). This effect is not undesirable in aphakic eyes since it alleviates the strong hyperopia of aphakia. That is the reason why many aphakic patients with silicone oil in the eye regard it as a disadvantage when the silicone oil is removed. If visual acuity makes it seem worthwhile, changes of refraction after silicone oil filling or removal should be considered and corrected.

## 2.1.2 Hypotheses On the Mode of Action of Silicone Oil

Concepts concerning the mode of action of silicone oil have changed constantly over the course of the years as a result of clinical experience and experimental studies. This process is not entirely finished: Whereas the hydraulic delamination of membranes from the retina took priority with Cibis, silicone oil nowadays is not used for this purpose at all. Some aspects of the mode of action of silicone oil are not entirely understood even today and are, accordingly, controversial. This aspect will be dealt with in detail in the discussion (Chap. 4). Therefore, only a short summary of the five concepts that comprise our present hypotheses on the mode of action of silicone oil is given here.

### 2.1.2.1 Tamponade

Silicone oil tamponades retinal defects of any size, anywhere, reliably and permanently due to its high surface tension. In a theoretical representation Petersen (1988b) convincingly demonstrated that silicone oil cannot flow under the retina if the distance between the retina and the pigment epithelium is small. The efficiency of the tamponade increases with decreasing distance (Fig. 2). Consequently, silicone oil can hold down an attached, traction-free retina very effectively. It is, however, not quite as well-suited to pressing down a detached retina.

Clinical experience confirms that a tension-free retina can be attached with silicone oil without problems, whereas silicone oil gets under the retina easily if tension persists. As a rule, renewed retinal detachments only occur in silicone filled eyes if the traction forces resulting from reproliferation of membranes exceed the tamponading power of the silicone oil.

In contrast to gas, the silicone bubble remains stable in the eye and thus keeps its tamponading effect permanently. This effective and reliable tamponade has two considerable advantages. Firstly, it allows the surgeon to carry out maneuvers which were either not possible or were limited out of fear of producing a retinal defect. Thus, we can now directly approach the retina surgically and remove epiretinal membranes thoroughly, a method which otherwise easily results in iatrogenic retinal tears. In view of the subsequent tamponade by silicone oil, retinotomies or retinectomies for the relief of traction, drainage of subretinal fluid, or removal of subretinal strands can now be performed safely. Secondly, reliable tamponade eliminates any rhegmatogenous components arising from redetachment of the retina. In eyes filled with liquid or gas, renewed formation of retinal tears can lead to a quick progression of redetachment. As the silicone tamponade limits the effect of newly formed tears, it can positively influence redetachments.

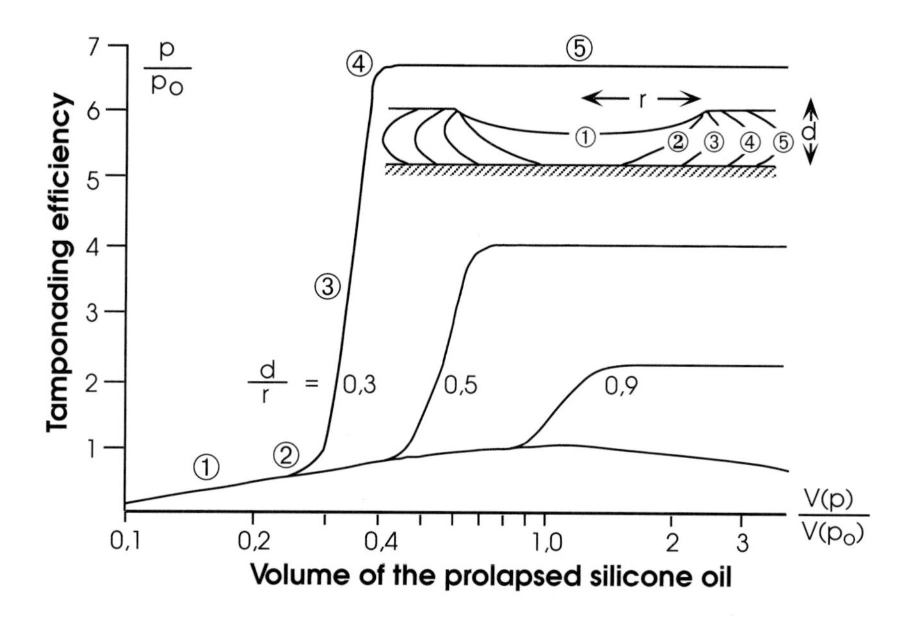


**Fig. 2.** Tamponading efficiency depends on retinal distance and defect size. The efficiency of the silicone oil tamponade increases with the decreasing distance of the retina from the pigment epithelium. If at a smaller distance the prolapsing silicone oil touches the pigment epithelium (②), it is compelled to take on a steeper surface curvature (③, ④ and ⑤). The surface tension, however, opposes this and thus produces a high tamponading pressure. The tamponading pressure attainable depends on the relation of the retinal distance (*d*) to the radius of the retinal defect (*r*). The smaller the distance or the bigger the defect, the more reliable is the tamponading effect. Consequently, for physical reasons, the oil can never get under an attached retina. (from: Petersen J. , 1988b)

### 2.1.2.2 "Space filler"

Due to the stability of the silicone oil bubble and its immiscibility with water, silicone oil limits the free movement of proliferative cells and biochemical mediators within the vitreous cavity (de Juan et al. 1986b, Chong et al. 1986). It creates, in fact, a new spatial compartmentalization in the eye. This effect probably modifies the intraocular proliferative process. The extent of reproliferation is limited hereby and a proliferative vitreoretinopathy perhaps prevented in susceptible eyes (Fastenberg et al. 1983, Gonvers 1983). Silicone oil can also change the growth characteristics of proliferative membranes leading to dense, flat, preretinal membranes, which we typically find in proliferative diabetic retinopathy, in the vitreous base, and along the edges of extensive retinectomies (see Color Plate 3, Fig 2a). Moreover, this "space filling" effect probably plays a part in the limitation of rubeosis iridis in proliferative diabetic retinopathy by physically inhibiting the diffusion of angiogenic mediators to the iris (de Juan et al. 1986b).

#### 2.1.2.3 Mechanical Inhibition of Membranous Contraction

Clinical experience has shown that redetachments of the retina by reproliferation or open defects happen less frequently and progress more slowly in eyes filled with silicone oil than in eyes that are not. This is probably due to elimination of the rhegmatogenous component in eyes with redetachment as described above, but mechanical forces probably play a part as well (Gonvers 1983, Lean et al. 1984). The stable form of the silicone bubble certainly does not prevent renewed proliferation, rather the traction forces are redirected parallel to the retina and can therefore exert less radial traction on it. Contraction of the membranes is thus counteracted. The concept of the modification of traction vectors by the intraocular silicone bubble is depicted in Fig. 3.

As a result of this effect redetachments with silicone oil are generally flat and confined to the periphery. The macula often remains attached for a long enough time, such that revision surgery can be planned without haste

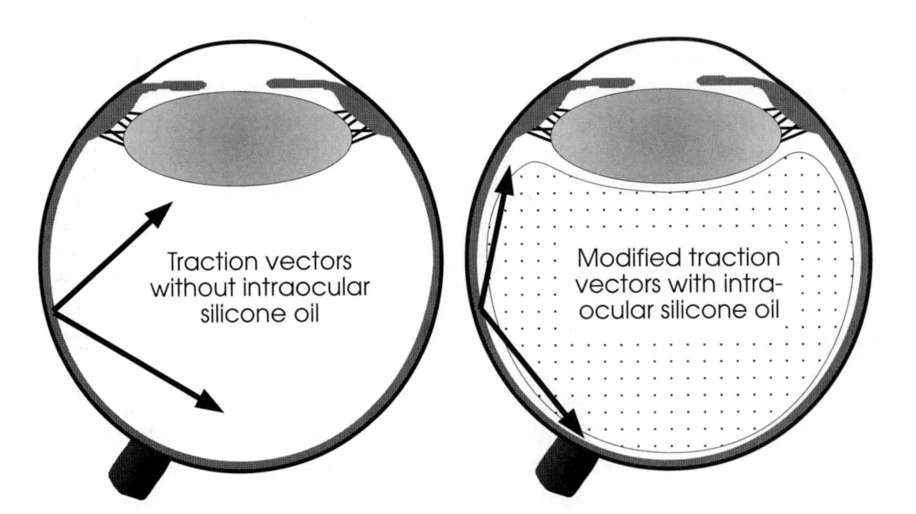


**Fig. 3.** Modification of traction vectors by the intraocular silicone bubble. Traction vectors are aligned parallel to the retina by the intraocular silicone bubble and can therefore exert less radial traction on the retina

and postponed if necessary until the general condition of the eye and the state of the proliferative process makes renewed surgery promising.

#### 2.1.2.4 Hemostasis

Silicone oil limits blood, fibrin, etc. to the space between the oil bubble and the retina. In doing so it also "tamponades" bleeding vessels and effectively limits or prevents secondary hemorrhages from diabetic vessels or retinal vessels along the edges of retinotomies. This effect is very welcome as blood and fibrin play an important part in the stimulation of proliferative processes (Miller et al. 1986b, de Juan et al. 1988). Moreover, the clear optics allow good postoperative supervision of the retinal situation, additional laser therapy if necessary, and, most of all, a quicker functional rehabilitation of the patient.

#### 2.1.2.5 Prophylaxis of Phthisis

It has been observed repeatedly that hypotonies tend to be less pronounced with silicone oil and that eyes tending to phthisis can sometimes be stabilized with silicone oil, at least temporarily; a shrinkage of the eye is thus counteracted. Due to the ensuing keratopathy, almost unavoidable in such eyes (see Sect. 3.3.2.5), this effect is not considered to be a primary indication for silicone oil injection.

The effects of silicone oil described above combine to result in a stabilization of the proliferative process. When this has subsided clinically and the retina is attached stably, the silicone oil can, in ideal circumstances, be removed.

## 2.2 Patients

### 2.2.1 Description of the Sample Investigated

This study comprises 483 eyes of 463 patients operated on with vitrectomy and silicone oil filling between April 1981 and January 1989 in Essen and Lübeck, FRG. Until March 1984 157 eyes were operated on in Essen; the remaining 326 eyes, from April 1984 onwards, in Lübeck. The operations were performed mainly by two surgeons: Horst Laqua (52.6%) and Klaus Lucke (44.1%). This group of patients is not identical to another one we have already reported on in cooperation with the Essen eye clinic, (Lucke et al. 1978a+b, Laqua et al. 1987) and in which very early cases without vitrectomy and, to a certain extent, also cases of other surgeons were included.

The indications for the use of silicone oil are relatively rare and such operations are consequently performed in specialized centers only. This results in a group of patients, of whom many come from a long distance with concomitant problems regarding postoperative care and control.

As a result of growing experience, the indications, techniques, instrumentation, and materials used have been subject to constant change over the course of the years. For the analysis of some special problems we have accordingly subdivided the total sample investigated into an early and a late group with a changeover on October 1, 1984. This date was chosen since routine silicone oil surgery was started in Lübeck then; since the patients operated on since then, as well as their data were, for logistic reasons, more easily accessible for this study; and since we started using the purified silicone oil OP5000 around that time. Of the eyes analyzed, 184 belonged to the early group, whereas the remaining 299 eyes of the late group comprised a sample operated on with techniques and materials that generally corresponded to present day conditions and should thus be representative of what can be achieved today.

The average age of the patients was 46 years, with a range from $1^1/_2$ to 84 years. There were 290 men (63%) and 173 women; the right eye was involved 254 times (53%), the left eye 229 times. In 125 of the 463 patients (27%) the contralateral eye was blind.

Of the 483 eyes, 236 (49%) had already been operated on previously once or several times, 122 (25%) were already aphakic, 16 (3%) were pseudophakic, 162 (34%) already had an encircling band, and 101 (21%) had previous vitreous surgery, 39 with intraocular air or gas injection.

## 2.2.2 Distribution of Indications

The diagnostic distribution of the 483 eyes is listed in Table 2. Due to considerable overlap, especially in patients with proliferative vitreoretinopathy, the indications for silicone oil surgery were broken down into a variety of subgroups to facilitate comparison and comprehension.

The most frequent indication was *proliferative vitreoretinopathy (PVR)*, and this was particularly true in the early phase of silicone oil surgery. PVR was somewhat less frequently represented in the late group (44%) than in the early group (52%) due to the fact that proliferative diabetic retinopathy (PDR) became a very frequent indication later on. Only PVR detachments not associated with giant tears, posterior holes, diabetes, or perforating trauma were defined as "uncomplicated". The classification of PVR into subgroups C1 – D3 was done in accordance with the classification of the

Retina Society (p. 38). Of the 144 eyes with uncomplicated PVR, 117 (81%) had already had retinal surgery once or several times, 45 (31%) were already aphakic,13 (9%) pseudophakic, 89 (62%) already had an encircling band, and 29 (20%) had undergone vitrectomy before, 15 with intraocular air or gas injection.

Giant tears and posterior holes could also be associated with perforating injuries or PVR and were therefore additionally subdivided into a total cohort and an "uncomplicated" one. Giant tears and posterior holes each comprised 15% of all patients, but for unknown reasons they were represented less in the late group (7% and 11%, respectively) than in the early group (27% and 20%, respectively).

Of the 45 uncomplicated *giant tears*, 26 (58%) had a size of 90°–170°, 12 (27%) of about 180°, and the remaining 7 (15%) 210° – 340°. A patient with 340° of tear actually had two giant tears of 170° each with small bridges at the 12 and 6 o'clock positions. In this same group 23 eyes were highly myopic, 3 had Marfan's syndrome, 2 a buphthalmos, 5 had suffered from blunt trauma, 3 had a congenital cataract, 3 a spontaneous lens luxation, and 6 an amblyopia; 4 of these eyes had already been operated on previously with buckling procedures.

Of 46 eyes with uncomplicated *posterior holes*, 36 were highly myopic and 17 aphakic. In this group 26 eyes had already been operated on previously with retinal surgery, 16 with an encircling band and 12 with vitrectomy and intraocular gas injection.

Of the 21 eyes with macular holes, 16 had a redetachment after previous vitreoretinal intervention, in the remaining 5 eyes silicone oil was used in the initial operation because the retina could not be flattened in a deep posterior staphyloma. Of the 16 eyes with previous surgery, 11 had a vitrectomy, 10 with intraocular gas; 4 had received an encircling band; and 1 a sponge explant. Here too, most of the eyes (16/21) were highly myopic and 7 were already aphakic.

In the early phase of silicone oil surgery we very rarely tackled operations involving patients with *PDR* since they are technically extremely difficult and we could thus expect disappointing results and serious complications. With growing experience and satisfying results the proportion of diabetic patients increased and this indication later became the predominant one.

Of the 136 diabetic eyes, 24 had already had previous vitreous surgery, 8 were aphakic, and 19 had a rubeosis iridis preoperatively. Of the 124 eyes in which silicone oil was used to tamponade retinal defects, 47 had retinal tears preoperatively; in the remaining eyes iatrogenic defects,, occurring at the time of surgery had to be tamponaded.

**Table 2.** Distribution of Indications for silicone oil surgery

| Indications | All patients *n* | All patients % | Early group *n* | Early group % | Late group *n* | Late group % |
|---|---|---|---|---|---|---|
| All diagnoses | 483 | 100.0 | 184 | 100.0 | 299 | 100.0 |
| PVR | 226 | 46.8 | 96 | 52.2 | 130 | 43.5 |
| without perforating injury [1] | 181 | 37.5 | 76 | 41.3 | 105 | 35.1 |
| with perforating injury | 45 | 9.3 | 20 | 10.9 | 25 | 8.4 |
| with giant tears | 20 | 4.1 | 15 | 8.2 | 5 | 1.7 |
| with posterior holes | 24 | 5.0 | 10 | 5.4 | 13 | 4.3 |
| Uncomplicated PVR | 144 | 29.8 | 55 | 29.9 | 89 | 29.8 |
| Stage C | 42 | 8.7 | 13 | 7.1 | 29 | 9.7 |
| C1 | 8 | 1.7 | 4 | 2.2 | 4 | 1.3 |
| C2 | 22 | 4.6 | 4 | 2.2 | 18 | 6.0 |
| C3 | 12 | 2.5 | 5 | 2.7 | 7 | 2.3 |
| Stage D | 102 | 21.1 | 42 | 22.8 | 60 | 20.1 |
| D1 | 27 | 5.6 | 13 | 7.1 | 14 | 4.7 |
| D2 | 58 | 12.0 | 22 | 12.0 | 36 | 12.0 |
| D3 | 17 | 3.5 | 7 | 3.8 | 10 | 3.3 |
| Giant tears | 70 | 14.5 | 49 | 26.6 | 21 | 7.0 |
| uncomplicated [1] | 45 | 9.3 | 30 | 16.3 | 15 | 5.0 |
| Posterior holes | 71 | 14.7 | 37 | 20.1 | 34 | 11.3 |
| uncomplicated [1] | 47 | 9.7 | 26 | 14.1 | 21 | 7.0 |
| MH uncomplicated | 21 | 4.3 | 12 | 6.5 | 9 | 3.0 |
| PDR[1] | 136 | 28.2 | 24 | 13.0 | 112 | 37.5 |
| with traction detachment | 124 | 25.7 | 17 | 9.2 | 107 | 35.8 |
| without traction detachment | 12 | 2.5 | 7 | 3.8 | 5 | 1.7 |
| Perforating Injury[1] | 61 | 12.6 | 26 | 14.1 | 35 | 11.7 |
| Miscellaneous Indications[1] | 13 | 2.7 | 2 | 1.1 | 11 | 3.7 |

PVR, proliferative vitreoretinopathy; MH, macular holes; PDR, proliferative diabetic retinopathy

[1]Sum total

The number of *perforating injuries* has remained constant over the years at 12%–14%. Although the overall frequency of perforating injuries has gone down in recent years this has been compensated for by the fact that the surgical possibilities have expanded and ever fewer patients are rejected as inoperable.

Of the 61 perforating injuries, 31 had already had previous vitreoretinal surgery, 20 times by vitrectomy, 10 times with an encircling band only, and 3 times with a sponge explant only. In addition 33 eyes were already aphakic and 12 still had one or several intraocular foreign bodies, which were removed at the time of silicone oil surgery.

"*Miscellaneous indications*" is a heterogeneous group of various complicated retinal problems, which do not fit into any of the above groups. In three patients we used silicone oil in situations involving multiple defects or defects difficult to identify without a typical PVR. One patient was highly myopic, had already been operated on several times without silicone oil, and it was not clear whether unidentified central or peripheral defects were responsible for the detachment. In the second patient there was probably a central defect in a large coloboma of the optic nerve. The third patient, who had a microphthalmos, had also been operated on unsuccessfully before and, at vitrectomy, showed an unusual form of vitreous contraction with a posterior retinal defect.

Four patients had an acute retinal necrosis with multiple retinal defects; another patient had an advanced age related maculopathy in her only eye, with massive subretinal hemorrhage which we tried to evacuate, and another patient had an advanced case of Coats' disease – also in the only eye – with massive peripheral neovascularization, subretinal exudates, and progressive phthisis.

On the whole the indication groups did not change much over the course of the years. Only PDR clearly came to the fore and finally represented about one third of all operations. This development and the present distribution of indications are similar to that of other groups active in silicone oil surgery.

## 2.3 Surgical Techniques

### 2.3.1 General

Encircling band, vitrectomy, membrane peeling, and coagulation are standard well-established techniques of conventional retinal and vitreous surgery and need not be described here (Machemer and Aaberg 1981, Schepens 1983, Michels 1981, Charles 1981).

We still place an equatorial *encircling band* in all eyes with PVR, giant tears, or perforating injuries. The aim of this measure is to: (a) Bring the periphery closer to the optical axis to facilitate vitrectomy in the vitreous base, (b) Counteract any contraction of the vitreous base postoperatively, and (c) Achieve delimitation of the posterior retina from the periphery by producing chorioretinal adhesion on the buckle edge with laser or cryotherapy. Closure of the tear is of secondary importance in silicone oil surgery.

Of the 483 patients, 162 already had encircling bands preoperatively. In 49 patients we revised the encircling band and in another 216 we applied a new one so that 378 patients (78%) finally had an encircling buckle. The great majority of the eyes without an encircling band either had a diabetic retinopathy with posterior traction detachment or had posterior holes.

Whereas in conventional retinal surgery the closure of more posterior retinal holes can only be achieved through additional *radial buckles*, this aspect has become insignificant in silicone oil surgery since tear closure can be achieved with silicone oil from the inside. Accordingly, the importance of such additional buckles to support holes posterior to the equator has decreased. Although we still applied such a buckle in 52 eyes (28%) in the early group, we considered it necessary in only 19 eyes (6%) in the late group.

The technique of *coagulation* has changed fundamentally in recent years due to the development of new technologies. At first only a cryoinstrument for external cryopexy was available, which we used in 192 eyes (40%). From June 1984 onwards it was complemented by an endocryoprobe (151 eyes, 31%), and in October 1987 an additional endolaser became available (79 eyes, 16%). In 107 eyes (22%) we performed additional postoperative argon laser coagulations.

## 2.3.2 Special Surgical Techniques for Various Indications

### 2.3.2.1 Proliferative Vitreoretinopathy

PVR consists of a posterior and an anterior component (Aaberg 1988), and in its surgery we proceed accordingly. A schematic diagram of the surgical procedure can be found in Fig. 4. An exemplary case is depicted in Color Plate 1, Figs. 1a + b.

The anterior component of PVR is characterized by shrinkage of the vitreous base and traction on the peripheral retina both anteriorly and towards the optical axis. In general, we therefore apply an equatorial encircling band in all eyes with PVR to counteract peripheral traction on the retina, and we also perform a thorough vitrectomy of the vitreous base (Fig. 4a). Epiretinal membrane peeling is carried out using the usual techniques (Fig. 4b) until the retina is completely mobilized. The subretinal fluid is drained with a flute needle through a posterior retinal defect (Fig. 4c), a paracentral drainage retinotomy, or through a peripheral tear with a "cannulated flute needle" (Flynn et al. 1988), while at the same time silicone oil is injected.

The posterior segment should be filled completely with silicone oil to achieve adequate tamponade and to minimize the recurrence of proliferation (see Color Plate 3, Figs 1a +b). When the retina is perfectly flat, the entire encircling buckle and any retinal defects or edges of retinectomies are coagulated with the endolaser (Fig. 4d) or treated with an external cryoprobe. If possible, cryopexy to the bare pigment epithelium of a tear is avoided, since this can result in dispersion of proliferative cells (Chignell et al. 1973, Campochiaro et al. 1985).

Hard to identify remnants of membranes, retinal shortening, subretinal strands, or peripheral vitreous contraction can be responsible for insufficient mobilization in spite of thorough membrane peeling. In eyes with peripheral vitreous contraction, we carried out an increasing number of circumferential peripheral relaxing cuts ("retinectomies"), sometimes up to 360°.

### 2.3.2.2 Giant Tears

As the retina in giant tears usually tends to fold over, surgery of giant tears can be divided into two basic steps: mobilization of the edge of the giant tear and fixation of the retinal edge in the anatomically correct position. A schematic diagram of the surgical procedure can be found in Fig. 5. An exemplary case is depicted in Color Plate 1, Figs. 2a + b.

We begin here too with an encircling band, as it supports the vitreous base in those areas of the peripheral retina that have not torn and coun-

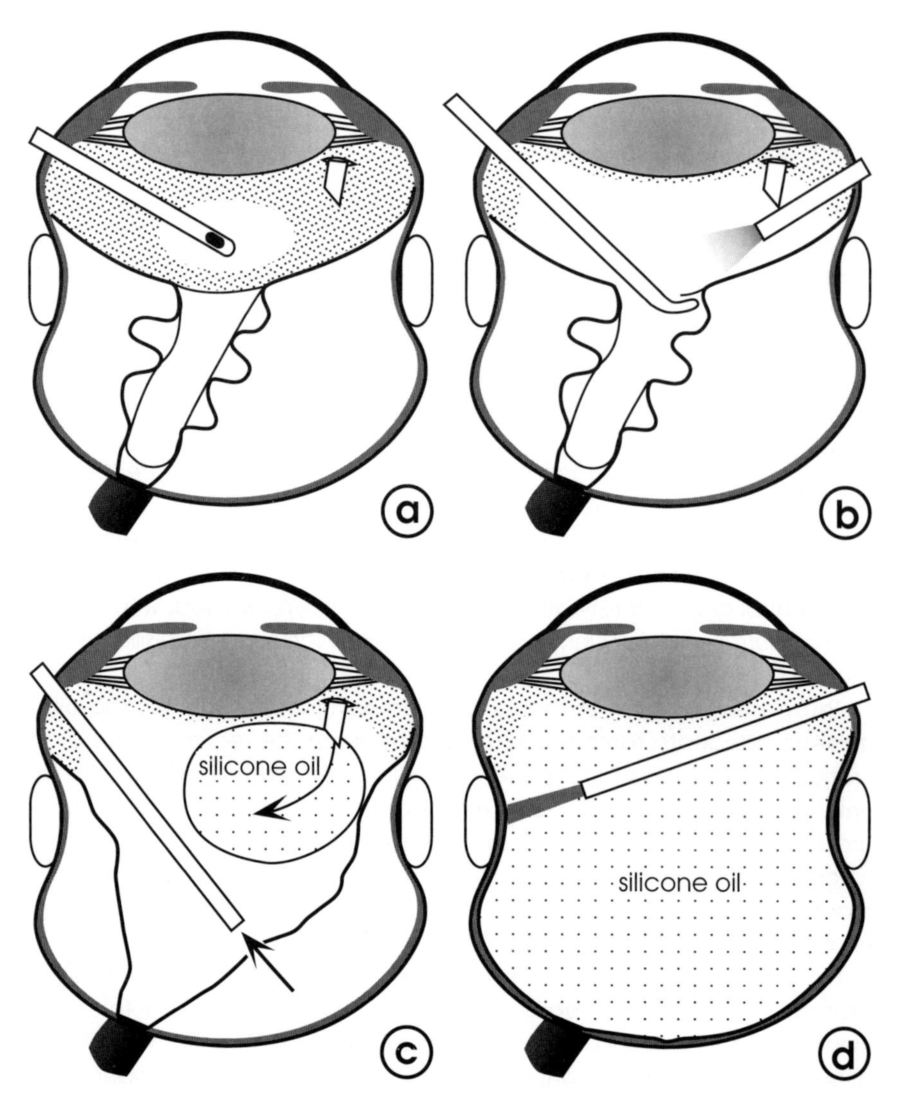


**Fig. 4a–d.** Surgical technique: PVR (proliferative vitreoretinopathy). For explanations see text. *Arrows* indicate direction of fluid movement

teracts the formation of a retinal tear and the subsequent development of a PVR as a result.

By thorough vitrectomy the retina can usually be mobilized without problems (Fig. 5a). The posterior edge of the giant tear itself is free of vitreous and residual traction is exerted on the remaining peripheral retinal remnants. This peripheral retina is removed as it is without function and the vitreous base attached to it could act as a scaffold for reproliferation. At

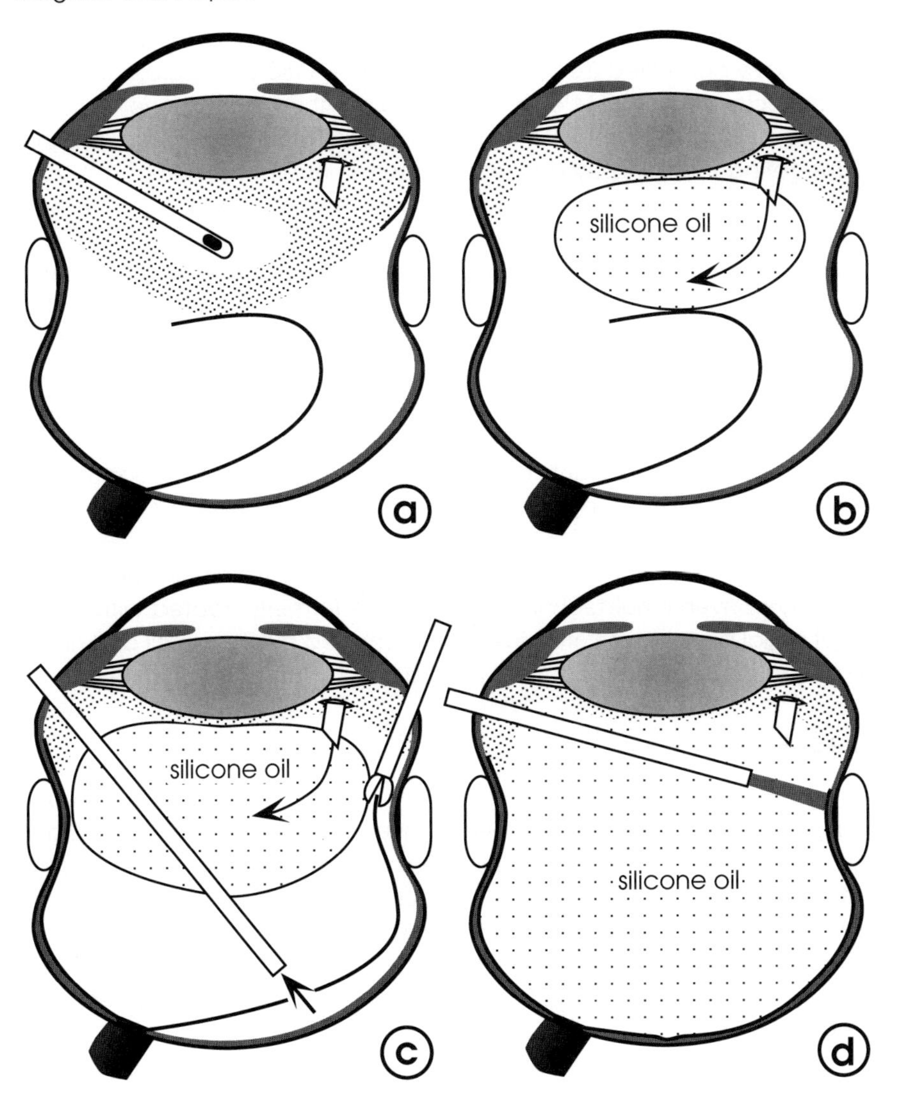


**Fig. 5a–d.** Surgical technique: giant tears. For explanations see text. *Arrows* indicate direction of fluid movement

the ends of the tears and in the periphery of the intact retina a particularly thorough vitrectomy is indicated as reproliferation leading to redetachment is most likely to occur here. Since giant tears carry a very high risk of developing into PVR, existing epiretinal membranes must be carefully searched for.

The retina can be unfolded with intraocular forceps or blunt instruments, but it tends to fold back again. Fixation of the retina in the anatomically correct position is technically very difficult, and many different techniques have been tried (see p. 88). From 1981 – 1983 we incarcerated the retina in sclerotomies in 14 eyes and found out then that silicone oil could be used as an instrument for the unfolding and, at the same time, fixation of the retina. Rotating tables, retinal sutures, incarcerations, and retinal tacks are hardly ever necessary and have not been used by us in recent years. The procedure is as follows:

While the retina is still folded over silicone oil is injected until the lower edge of the silicone oil bubble reaches the encircling buckle (Fig. 5b). The retina then is folded back with forceps or a blunt instrument and pulled between the silicone oil and the pigment epithelium (Fig. 5c) where it is held by the surface tension of the silicone oil. Injection of the oil is resumed and the subretinal fluid drained through a small drainage retinotomy. Finally the edge of the giant tear is sealed off by endolaser coagulation (Fig. 5d), and the encircling buckle in the remaining quadrants is treated by cryopexy or endolaser.

Radial extensions at the corners of giant tears, which are difficult to close by conventional techniques and were formerly treated with additional radial buckles, are effectively tamponaded by silicone oil and need no further support. They too are simply sealed by laser coagulation.

#### 2.3.2.3 Posterior Holes

Macular holes can usually be successfully attached with the method described by Gonvers and Machemer (Gonvers 1982b, Laqua 1985) and, accordingly, vitrectomy with gas injection is our therapy of choice in this situation. Only complicated posterior retinal holes provide indications for the use of silicone oil. These indications are: (a) conus defects and defects in areas of chorioretinal degeneration (Color Plate 1, Figs. 3a + b); (b) posterior holes associated with PVR; and (c) redetachments after vitrectomy and gas filling.

A schematic diagram of the surgical procedure can be found in Fig. 6. With posterior holes an encircling band is usually not necessary unless PVR is present. After vitrectomy (Fig. 6a) and separation of possible adhesions between central retina and vitreous or peeling of thin preretinal membranes (Fig. 6b) which frequently exist, the eye is filled with silicone oil (Fig. 6c) under simultaneous endodrainage with a flute needle. The edges of the defects are then coagulated (Fig. 6d).

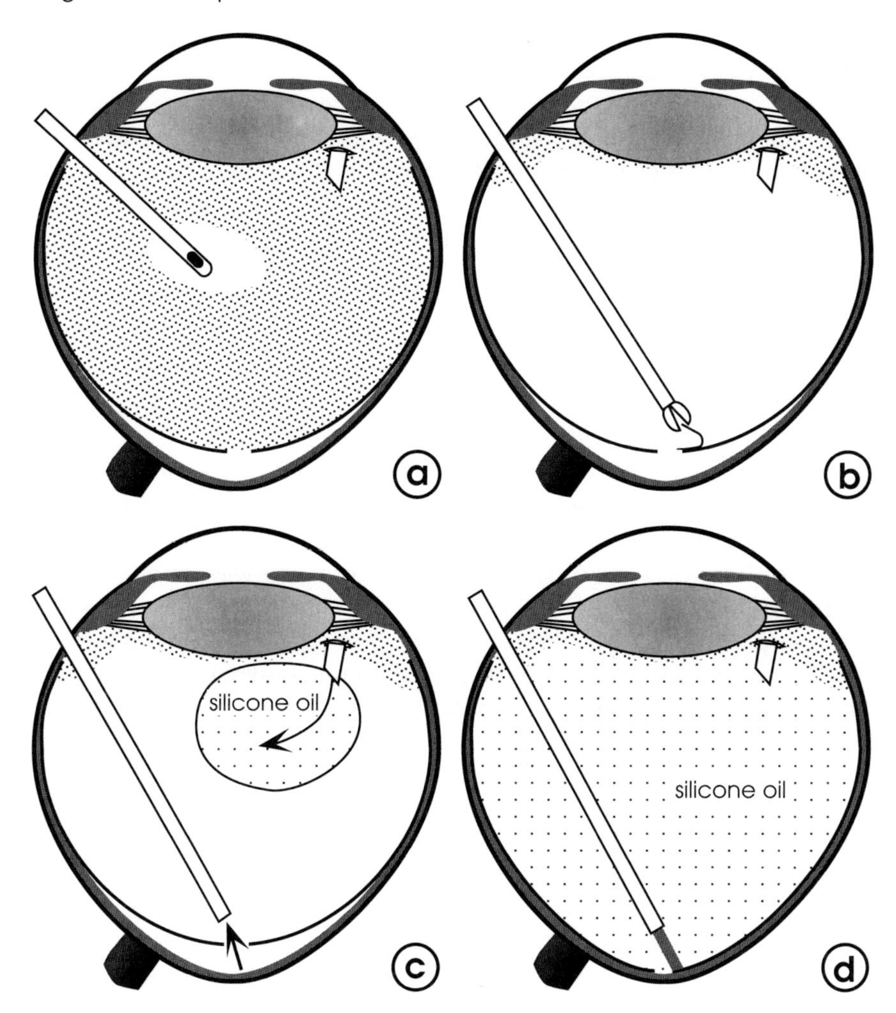


**Fig. 6a–d.** Surgical technique: posterior holes. For explanations see text. *Arrows* indicate direction of fluid movement

### 2.3.2.4 Proliferative Diabetic Retinopathy

The surgical problems of eyes with progressive PDR differ considerably from those with other indications. Thick preretinal membranes, which are often heavily vascularized, constitute the main difficulty. They span the posterior pole and adhere firmly to the disc and other points along the major retinal vessels.

In "burnt out" PDR, where the membranes are completely atrophic and it is usually not necessary to use silicone oil, careful segmentation of these membranes is often sufficient. Small remnants can be left as long as traction on the retina is completely relieved.

In most advanced PDRs with traction detachment the proliferations are interspersed with blood carrying vessels and should be completely removed. Many of these eyes already have retinal defects caused by traction. In addition injury of the retina during membrane separation is often unavoidable; in these cases we use silicone oil to tamponade retinal defects. A schematic diagram of the surgical procedure can be found in Fig. 7.

As long as the pathology is restricted to the posterior pole, we can usually do without an encircling band. Due to the danger of rubeosis iridis developing postoperatively, we attempt to preserve the lens as often as possible unless cataract obstructs the view during surgery.

After removal of the vitreous (Fig. 7a), the space between the retina and the proliferative tissue is accessed, the membranes are undermined with blunt instruments, and the attachments between proliferations and retinal vessels are severed by blunt dissection or cut with intraocular microscissors (Fig. 7b). For better hemostasis it is important to sever the proliferations close to the retinal vessels rather than cut somewhat distant from them. If proliferative vessels are separated from the retinal vessels by blunt dissection, bleeding can be kept to a minimum.

In particularly difficult situations where bleeding cannot be controlled, thrombin can be added to the infusion line (de Bustros et al. 1985). In doing so bleeding is not entirely prevented but tends to stop more quickly. Unfortunately, thrombin may lead to a severe inflammatory reaction postoperatively, we have therefore used it only five times in the last 2 years.

The aim of surgery is the complete removal of *all* proliferative membranes; otherwise very aggressive reproliferations can develop under silicone oil. Proliferations on the optic disc should also be removed and can easily be pulled off with intraocular forceps. Surprisingly, this causes no problems and practically never results in severe bleeding.

In eyes with incomplete posterior vitreous detachment, occasionally thick proliferative membranes exist that are firmly adherent to a retina which has already been detached for some time and is, accordingly, thin and atrophic. In such situations it is sometimes impossible to separate the proliferations from the retina and we must resort to retinectomy (see Color Plate 2, Figs. 2a + b). This has proved necessary in 34 of our 124 eyes (27%) with PDR and traction detachment.

When the retina is free of traction, it must be thoroughly cleared of remnants of blood as they may constitute a stimulus for renewed preretinal proliferation. Silicone oil can then be injected in the usual way (Fig. 7c). Subretinal fluid is usually drained with the flute needle through preexisting holes or defects that develop intraoperatively.

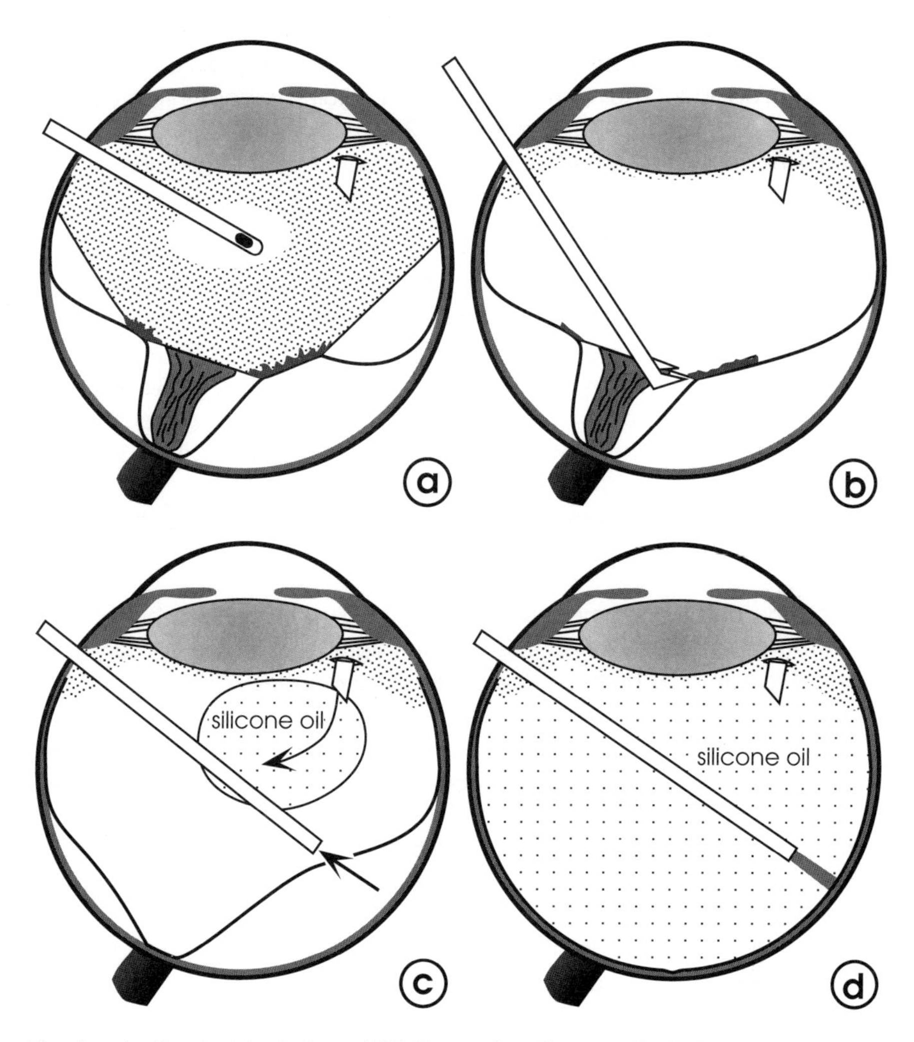


**Fig. 7a–d.** Surgical technique: PDR. For explanations see text. *Arrows* indicate direction of fluid movement

Finally, all retinal defects are surrounded by endolaser coagulation and a disseminated panretinal laser coagulation is carried out (Fig. 7d).

Due to the excellent "hemostatic" properties of silicone oil, we used it in 12 eyes with PDR without retinal holes or detachment. These included eight eyes with very active proliferations, in which we expected massive and recurrent postoperative hemorrhages unless we filled the eyes with silicone oil, thereby using it for faster visual rehabilitation and the prevention of rubeosis. Two more eyes had already been operated on without silicone oil and bled recurrently. We also used silicone oil in two young female diabetics whose proliferations were so massively vascularized that we employed silicone oil primarily to guard against rubeosis iridis (an exemplary case is depicted in Color Plate 2, Figs. 1a + b). In all patients silicone oil instillation facilitated early and extensive laser coagulation.

#### 2.3.2.5 Perforating Injuries

For all practical purposes, perforating injuries behave like fulminant PVR, and correspondingly the surgical principles (encircling band, vitrectomy, peripheral and central membrane peeling, silicone oil) apply to both clinical pictures (for an exemplary case see Color Plate 2, Figs. 3a + b). As anatomical situation and surgical procedure in perforating trauma are highly variable it is not feasible to depict a representative surgical scheme.

In addition to PVR several additional potential problems should be mentioned with respect to perforating injuries:

1. Since the anterior segment is frequently involved, considerable *optical obstacles* to surgery often exist. These might necessitate primary pars plana lensectomy or, if the cornea is badly clouded, a temporary keratoprosthesis with subsequent penetrating keratoplasty.
2. In recent injuries massive *intraocular hemorrhages* can occur intraoperatively, which, by themselves, can thwart surgical success. This aspect is dealt with in Chap. 4.
3. Incarcerated *intraocular foreign bodies* must be removed; however, doing so can also result in massive and virtually uncontrollable hemorrhages.
4. Retinal and choroidal injuries caused by foreign bodies are sources of *massive proliferations* and the retina is often pulled into such wounds. It is therefore important to free the vicinity of such wounds thoroughly of vitreous and blood.
5. If the *retina* is already being *pulled into* such a *wound*, there is no chance of permanent reattachment unless the retina is cut around the incarceration site. This also carries a considerable risk of uncontrollable hemorrhage. The incarceration site and retinal edges should thus be sealed off broadly with the endolaser.

## 2.3.3 Special Techniques

### 2.3.3.1 Lens Extraction

Lens extraction may be required if a cataract interferes optically or if it is necessary to treat the peripheral vitreous and a clear lens is in the way.

In the context of vitreous surgery the decision as to what technique of lens extraction to use is not always an easy one to make. Whether to use intracapsular or extracapsular extraction with phakoemulsification or nuclear expression or, alternatively, the pars plana approach with a fragmatome must be decided from case to case depending on the initial situation, equipment available, and the particular skills of the surgeon.

We generally prefer the approach via the pars plana as it does not stress the anterior segment and thus does not endanger a good view to the posterior segment. Furthermore, it does not result in large corneoscleral wounds, which could make vitreoretinal maneuvers difficult or impossible due to the danger of wound dehiscence.

If a cataract exists before the beginning of vitreous surgery, the lens is removed via the pars plana at the start of the operation. The pars plana approach is also useful in revision surgery when the lens has to be removed and surgery must be continued in the posterior segment. In most cases, when we wanted to remove the lens and the silicone oil in one procedure, we also removed the lens via the pars plana.

Lately, we have considered the implantation of an intraocular lens after silicone oil removal. For this purpose we sometimes use a two-step procedure since ultrasound biometry cannot be reliably performed in eyes filled with silicone (Shugar et al. 1986). We remove the silicone oil in the first step, leaving the cataract. In a second operation a few weeks later a normal extracapsular cataract extraction with posterior chamber lens implantation can be performed. Alternatively, we remove the silicone oil and the lens via the pars plana leaving the capsular ring intact. If needed, a posterior chamber lens can be implanted into the ciliary sulcus at some later date.

### 2.3.3.2 Silicone Oil Injection and Drainage of Subretinal Fluid

Silicone oil is injected via the standard infusion line (Fig. 4c). Since we use highly viscous oil exclusively, we prefer manual injection systems to automatic pumps (Fig. 8a), which are too slow with these oils. We either use resterilizable glass syringes with a threaded plunger (Fig. 8b) or 10 ml standard plastic syringes with a Luer-Lok, which are inserted in a holder with a screw mechanism (Fig. 8c).

During silicone oil injection, pre- and subretinal fluid is evacuated through the flute needle. External drainage through the sclera is hardly ever used nowadays because of the high risk of complications (choroidal detachment, subretinal bleeding). In the early group we drained 119 times internally and 86 times externally (21 times both techniques) and have used the external technique only 5 times since October 1984.

Since it allows a perfect view to the whole fundus, we always perform silicone oil injection under binocular ophthalmoscope observation or the binocular indirect operating microscope ("BIOM", Spitznas 1987) and always exchange silicone oil for fluid. To avoid dangerously high intraocular pressures, we ensure that the point of the flute needle stays in the fluid compartment throughout the maneuver. The interface between silicone oil and fluid phase is visible as a ring on the flute needle and this serves as

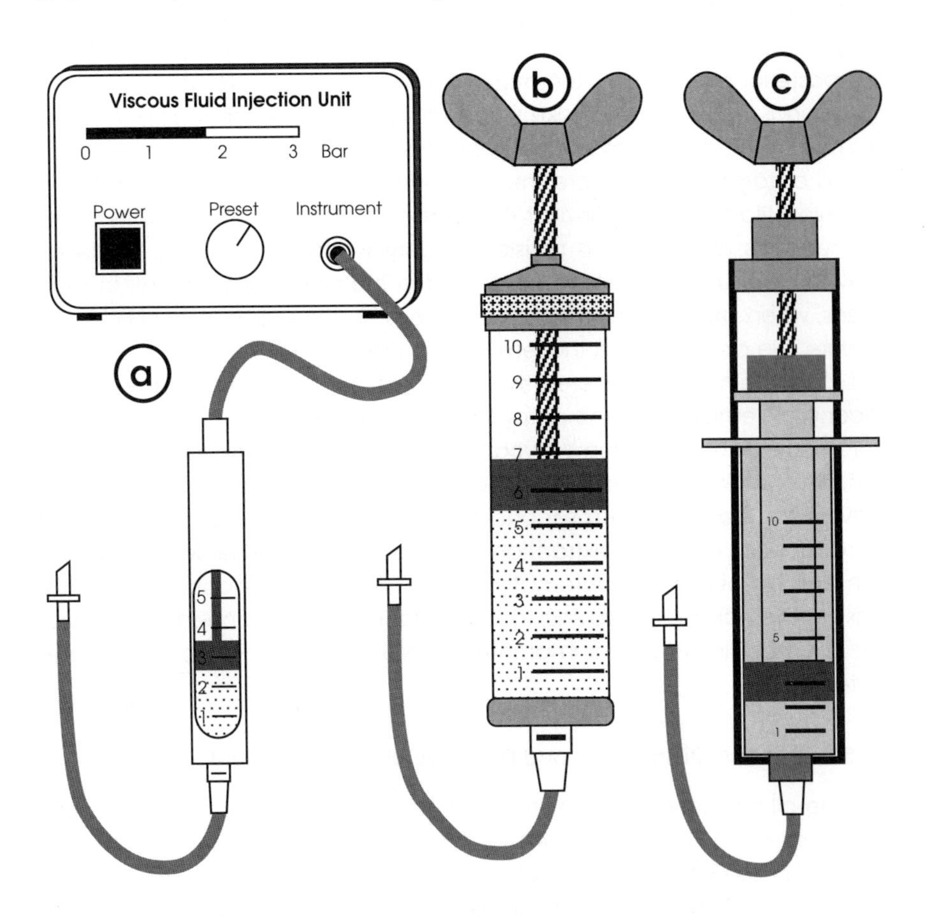


**Fig. 8a–c.** Systems for the injection of silicone oil. ⓐ automatic pump, ⓑ threaded glass-syringe, ⓒ holder for plastic syringes

an indicator of the level of oil filling.

We prefer the exchange of silicone oil for fluid to that of silicone oil for air which is practiced widely in the USA. The proponents of silicone-air exchange believe that they can better identify remaining traction; however, the view of the fundus during the procedure is considerably worse, and this results in inferior control of the maneuver. Furthermore, direct manipulations of the retina (e.g., folding back of a rolled over retinal edge, p. 23) are impossible. A decisive advantage of silicone oil surgery, which should not to be underestimated, is thus not taken advantage of.

#### 2.3.3.3 Retinotomy and Retinectomy

Cutting retina is done in order to drain subretinal fluid or relieve traction. The concept of actually incising retina is perhaps the most revolutionary of this surgery and has definitely been responsible for the name "extreme vitreoretinal surgery". It requires all retinal surgeons to overcome considerable psychological barriers. Cutting of the retina, is, however, often a decisive step in its mobilization (for an exemplary case see Color Plate 2, Figs. 3a + b).

Smaller central retinotomies, for the removal of subretinal fluid or subretinal strands, can most easily be produced by high power endodiathermy. For drainage an area should be chosen that is relatively posterior but outside the vascular arcs and not too close to larger vessels. Defects in the visual field can be minimized if a spot in the temporal upper quadrant (lower nasal visual field) or temporally in the raphe is chosen.

Longer retinal incisions can be performed either with sharp instruments (intraocular scissors, vitrectomy probe) after initial diathermy to the area or with diathermy directly. We generally prefer the diathermy instrument at a high power setting since by this method we can achieve more reliable hemostasis.

Peripheral retinal remnants are without function and should be removed. Since we therefore remove larger areas of retina when we make long incisions, we prefer to refer to such incisions as "retinectomies".

#### 2.3.3.4 Silicone Oil Removal

Cibis and Scott regarded silicone oil as a permanent tamponade which need not be removed from the eye again. Today the generally accepted trend, originally propagated by Gonvers (1985), is to remove the silicone oil from the eye if possible.

There are different systems for silicone oil removal of different technical complexity, ranging from special cannulas to electronically controlled automatic drainage pumps. In practice, the more complex systems have not proved to be very useful, especially with more viscous oils. The most

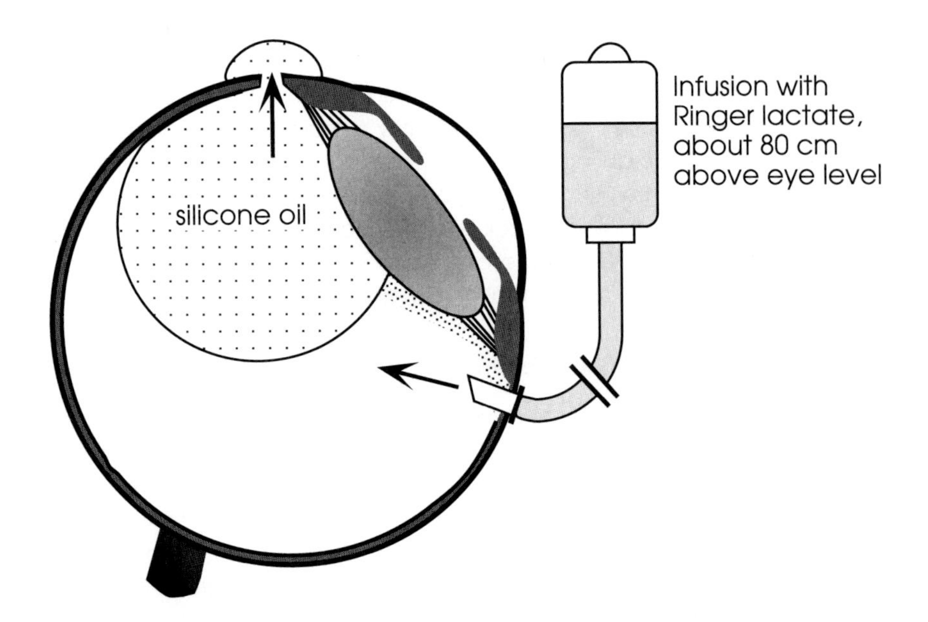


**Fig. 9.** Technique of silicone oil removal. For explanations see text. *Arrows* indicate direction of fluid movement

simple method is still passive drainage of the silicone oil by a slightly enlarged pars plana sclerotomy. A scheme of the procedure is shown in Fig. 9.

For silicone oil removal we suture an infusion port into the lower temporal pars plana as in a normal vitrectomy. We then make a pars plana sclerotomy of about 1.5-2 mm in the temporal upper quadrant and lift the infusion bottle to a height of about 80-100 cm above eye level (about 60-75 mmHg intraocular pressure). The eye is turned so that the sclerotomy is the highest point of the eye and spread the incision slightly with microforceps. We then wait until the silicone oil has drained from the eye by infusion pressure alone. The process takes about 10 – 20 min depending on the size of the incision. Alternatively, the silicone oil can also be withdrawn from the eye with a normal 10 ml syringe and a 1 mm cannula with a specially wide bore. By repeated liquid-gas exchange most of the remaining small silicone oil droplets can subsequently be mobilized and removed from the eye.

#### 2.3.3.5 Inferior Basal Iridectomy ("Ando Iridectomy")

The anterior chamber should at all times be free of silicone oil in order to reduce the risk of keratopathy and to avoid early angle-closure glaucoma. For this purpose a basal iridectomy at the 6 o'clock meridian, first

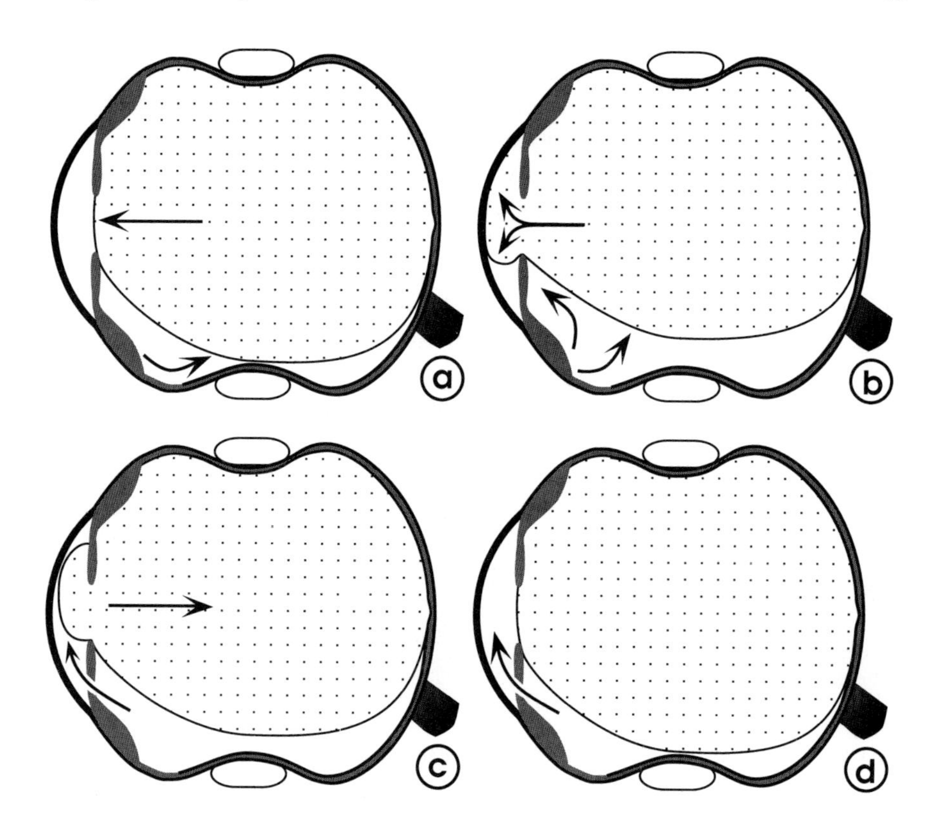


**Fig. 10a–d.** Action of the inferior basal iridectomy. For explanations see text. *Arrows* indicate direction of fluid movement

described by Ando (1987), has proved successful, and we have used it in all aphakic eyes since October 1984. Its action is described in Fig. 10.

Silicone oil in an eye rises to the top due to its specific weight, which is lower than water, whereas the aqueous humor produced by the ciliary body collects in the lower part of the eye and presses the silicone oil bubble further up. In aphakic eyes this can lead to pupillary-block (Fig. 10a). The oil is eventually pushed into the anterior chamber through the pupil, and this results in secondary angle closure (Fig. 10b). If, however, an iridectomy is made at 6 o'clock, the aqueous humor can flow into the anterior chamber directly and push the silicone oil back behind the pupillary plane (Fig. 10d).

The inferior basal iridectomy is cut with the vitreous cutter into the iris from behind; this is done towards the end of the operation just before the silicone oil is injected.

The Ando iridectomy can spontaneously close up again through fibrin formation and reproliferation. It is important therefore to make it large enough and to remove all material behind the iris that could constitute a scaffold for reproliferation (capsular remnants, peripheral vitreous). If the iridectomy is closed, silicone oil will prolapse into the anterior chamber, and pupillary-block as well as angle-closure could result in a massive increase in intraocular pressure. In that case the iridectomy must be reopened immediately as a matter of urgency. This can usually be performed easily with the pulsed Nd: YAG laser, which we have used successfully 15 times in 156 iridectomies. When the iridectomy is reopened, aqueous humor flows into the anterior chamber immediately, and the silicone oil retreats behind the pupillary plane within minutes (see Color Plate 4, Figs. 1a + b).

## 2.4 Statistical Method

### 2.4.1 Clinical Examinations and Observation Intervals

Preoperatively, all patients underwent a basic ophthalmologic examination including tests of visual acuity, intraocular pressure, slit-lamp examination, and binocular indirect ophthalmoscopy. If indicated, gonioscopy, ultrasound, and visual field examination and photo documentation were performed as well.

After discharge the patients were reexamined at regular intervals. For this study clinical data obtained after 3, 6, 12, and 24 months and thereafter in yearly intervals were made use of. Examinations were scheduled more frequently if necessitated by complications. If patients did not appear for control visits, the attending ophthalmologists were asked for a written report.

All data were entered into a data base which was up-dated continuously. Data collection was terminated on February 28, 1989.

As many of our patients came from afar, it was impossible to achieve a 100% follow-up. In spite of all efforts on our part, some of our patients either did not appear for follow-up visits or else information from the ophthalmologists was unobtainable. In 23 patients (5%) long-term follow-up was impossible on account of death or enucleation of the operated eye (11 times). In all, 83% of the eyes in the study were followed up postoperatively for at least 6 months. The average length of follow-up was 21.7 months.

The results after a follow-up period of 6 months are generally considered in ophthalmology, particularly in vitreoretinal surgery, as an acceptable end point. An 83% follow-up rate at 6 months is not unusual in the literature and is widely accepted. We have tried, however, to examine our patients after even longer intervals because of the particular long-term problems of silicone oil surgery. After 24 months only 53% of the patients returned for follow-up examinations. Our explanations for this low rate are:

1. many patients with redetachment did not return for regular examinations and neither did patients with an attached retina and the silicone oil successfully removed.
2. The 24 month follow-up period was not completed.
3. For those patients coming from afar, with long journeys involved, such long time controls were not reasonable.

To be able to make reliable statistical statements after such a long period of time in a cohort of ever decreasing size, a statistical process such as life table analysis was required.

### 2.4.2 Life Table Analysis

The life table method of Cutler and Ederer (1958) was chosen; this is a biometric method for indirect comparison of survival rates in cohorts of different lengths of observation, which was originally developed for statistical evaluation of cancer patients. Life table analysis has established itself in the analysis of cohorts with different lengths of follow-up (Ederer 1973) and has the advantage that every patient is considered, independent of the length of observation. This method is based on simple mathematical formulae which can be applied even without specialized mathematical knowledge.

To apply the life table method to this analysis, an assumption had, however, to be made. Normally, with cancer statistics, all patients are alive at the beginning of the observation period. Analogously, all our patients should have attached retinas at the time of the first observation interval. If directly applied, life table analysis would be suitable for stating which percentage of the primarily successful operated on eyes had an attached retina at the end of the observation period. To facilitate comparison with other surgical statistics, however, it was more important to know how many of the operated on patients could be considered successes after a specified period of observation. For the first observation interval, a hypothetical point of time during the initial operation was therefore chosen for which it was assumed that at this point in time all eyes had attached retinas. If this premise was used, life table analysis was applicable to our purpose.

For an automatized analysis we wrote a simple computer program in Basic, by means of which each chosen subcohort or the whole data set could be examined with respect to various parameters.

The following was calculated by the program:

1. Anatomic results absolutely and cumulatively (life table)
2. Improvements in visual acuity absolutely and cumulatively
3. Cumulative portion of patients with preserved ambulatory vision
4. Average visual acuity
5. Glaucoma rate absolutely and cumulatively
6. Keratopathy rate absolutely and cumulatively
7. Average length of observation

In addition the program automatically produced a scatter graph of the preoperative and postoperative visual acuities (Fig. 13).

In the interest of clarity we omitted standard deviations in many instances in the graphic representations unless they were essential for making a particular point. The groups examined were subdivided according to clinical criteria and were not randomized. We therefore did not include calculations of significance in comparative representations (Figs. 17, 18, 25–31).

## 2.4.3 Definitions

### 2.4.3.1 Anatomic Success

Criteria for the definition of anatomic success after retinal surgery were laid down by the international conference of the Retina Foundation and were defined as completely attached retina posterior to the encircling buckle. This definition is well-established and was adopted for the purpose of this study. For patients with eyes that had no encircling band, attachment of the peripheral retina was also included in the definition of success.

### 2.4.3.2 Visual Success

The Retina Foundation defined visual success as a postoperative improvement of visual acuity over the preoperative state. It later became accepted that such an improvement should correspond to a doubling of the spatial resolution.

**Table 3.** Definition of visual acuity groups

| Group | Visual acuity | |
|---|---|---|
| 8 | 1.2 – 0.8 | (20/16 – 20/25) |
| 7 | 0.7 – 0.4 | (20/32 – 20/50) |
| 6 | 0.3 – 0.2 | (20/63 – 20/100) |
| 5 | 0.15 – 0.1 | (20/125 – 20/200) |
| 4 | 0.05 – 1/25 | (20/400 – 20/500) |
| 3 | 1/35 – 1/50 | (20/700 – 20/1000) |
| 2 | counting fingers/hand movement | |
| 1 | light perception | |
| 0 | no light perception | |

To simplify data analysis, visual acuities were graded in nine steps. The step from one group to the next higher one was logarithmical (at least in the higher groups) and was equal to a doubling of spatial resolution. The subdivision in the lower groups proved useful in practice. The various visual acuity groups are defined in Table 3. Visual success was defined as improving from one group to the next higher one.

### 2.4.3.3 Preservation of Ambulatory Vision (Average Visual Acuity)

In eyes such as those reported on in this study the evaluation of "visual success" as defined above was not a true reflection of genuine functional success. A giant tear with the macula still attached, a preoperative visual acuity of 0.7, and a postoperative visual acuity of 0.6 would by this definition not have been considered a functional success. The natural course without surgery would, however, lead to loss of vision such that preserving a visual acuity of 0.6 or even 0.1 should by rights be regarded as a success. For this reason we evaluated the functional results also on the basis of another criterion which does more justice to the clinical pictures discussed here: In a second analysis of visual results the percentage of eyes in which ambulatory vision, defined as a visual acuity of 1/50 (20/1000) or better, could be preserved was evaluated.

In order to determine general trends in the changes of visual performance in groups of patients, an average visual acuity was calculated mathematically on the basis of the frequency of the various visual groups present within the cohort. This average visual acuity was used for the evaluation of silicone oil toxicity.

### 2.4.3.4 Classification of PVR Stages

PVR was classified according to the system established by the terminology committee of the Retina Society (1983). It is summarized in Table 4.

**Table 4.** Classification of PVR

| Grade | Definition |
|---|---|
| A | Vitreous haze, vitreous pigment clumps |
| B | Wrinkling of the inner retinal surface, rolled edge of Retinal break, retinal stiffness, vessel tortuosity |
| C | Full thickness fixed retinal folds |
| C1 | In one quadrant |
| C2 | In two quadrants |
| C3 | In three quadrants |
| D | Full thickness fixed retinal folds in four quadrants |
| D1 | Wide funnel shape |
| D2 | Narrow funnel shape (fills a 20D lens) |
| D3 | Closed funnel (optic nerve head not visible) |

# 3 Results

## 3.1 Anatomic and Functional Results

Table 5 shows the results for anatomic and functional success by direct analysis (successes at the end of the observation time) for the indication groups described in Sect. 2.2.3. The corresponding results by life table analysis can be found in Table 6.

For the sake of completeness analogous tables for the results of the early group (Tables A and B) and the late group (Tables C and D) can be found in the Appendix.

In the tables the values at 6 and 24 months are represented exemplarily, since the results at 6 months are usually reported by convention and since in almost all life table analyses a stabilization of the values occurred by 24 months so that these values could be regarded as final results. Although we did calculate life table values beyond 24 months for many indication groups, they were often not very significant since the numbers of patients in the cohorts were too small; they are therefore not reported.

In the second lines of Table 5 and 6 those results are listed that one arrives at if all patients with a follow-up of less than 6 months would be left out of the analysis as is frequently done in other studies. Our results under those circumstances generally turned out to be better by a few percentage points than if the whole sample was analyzed. From this it could be deduced that there was a higher proportion of failures among patients with only a short observation period. The fact that we included those patients in our analysis might therefore have changed the results slightly for the *worse*, if at all, however, this should have been neutralized to a large extent by use of life table analysis. Conversely, an elimination of those patients would have falsified the results inadmissibly for the *better*.

**Table 5.** Absolute anatomic and functional successes at the end of follow-up (all eyes)

| Diagnosis | *n* | Successes at the end of follow-up | | | | | | Follow-up (months) |
|---|---|---|---|---|---|---|---|---|
| | | Anatomical | | Visual | | Visual acuity ≥1/50 | | |
| | | *n* | % | *n* | % | *n* | % | |
| All diagnoses | 483 | 350 | 72.5 | 283 | 58.6 | 313 | 64.8 | 21.7 |
| ≥ 6 mos. follow-up | 400 | 293 | 73.3 | 248 | 62.0 | 270 | 67.5 | 25.7 |
| PVR, total | 226 | 152 | 67.3 | 131 | 58.0 | 145 | 64.2 | 22.3 |
| without perforating injury | 181 | 128 | 70.7 | 107 | 59.1 | 121 | 66.9 | 23.1 |
| with perforating injury | 45 | 24 | 53.3 | 24 | 53.3 | 24 | 53.3 | 19.2 |
| with giant tears | 20 | 11 | 55.0 | 6 | 30.0 | 10 | 50.0 | 22.7 |
| with posterior holes | 23 | 16 | 69.6 | 12 | 52.2 | 14 | 60.9 | 24.8 |
| PVR, uncomplicated | 144 | 103 | 71.5 | 91 | 63.2 | 100 | 69.4 | 22.6 |
| Stage C | 42 | 32 | 76.2 | 23 | 54.8 | 31 | 73.8 | 20.0 |
| Stage C1 | 8 | 7 | 87.5 | 6 | 75.0 | 7 | 87.5 | 23.8 |
| Stage C2 | 22 | 17 | 77.3 | 14 | 63.6 | 17 | 77.3 | 17.0 |
| Stage C3 | 12 | 8 | 66.7 | 3 | 25.0 | 7 | 58.3 | 23.0 |
| Stage D | 102 | 71 | 69.6 | 68 | 66.7 | 69 | 67.6 | 23.6 |
| Stage D1 | 27 | 24 | 88.9 | 21 | 77.8 | 22 | 81.5 | 30.1 |
| Stage D2 | 58 | 35 | 60.3 | 35 | 60.3 | 36 | 62.1 | 21.6 |
| Stage D3 | 17 | 12 | 70.6 | 12 | 70.6 | 11 | 64.7 | 20.2 |
| Giant tears, total | 70 | 58 | 82.9 | 43 | 61.4 | 49 | 70.0 | 24.1 |
| uncomplicated | 45 | 42 | 93.3 | 32 | 71.1 | 34 | 75.6 | 24.6 |
| Posterior holes, total | 71 | 56 | 78.9 | 46 | 64.8 | 51 | 71.8 | 23.6 |
| uncomplicated | 47 | 40 | 85.1 | 34 | 72.3 | 37 | 78.7 | 22.6 |
| MH, uncomplicated | 21 | 20 | 95.2 | 15 | 71.4 | 18 | 85.7 | 19.8 |
| PDR, total | 136 | 96 | 73.0 | 73 | 53.7 | 82 | 60.3 | 19.5 |
| with detachment | 124 | 86 | 69.4 | 64 | 51.6 | 73 | 58.9 | 19.0 |
| without detachment | 12 | 10 | 83.3 | 9 | 75.0 | 9 | 75.0 | 24.5 |
| Perforating injury, total | 61 | 37 | 60.7 | 35 | 57.4 | 35 | 57.4 | 19.3 |
| Other diagnoses | 13 | 7 | 53.8 | 2 | 15.4 | 4 | 30.1 | 24.2 |

PVR, proliferative vitreoretinopathy; MH, macular hole; PDR, proliferative diabetic retinopathy

**Table 6.** Anatomic and functional successes after 6 and 24 months by life table analysis[1] (all eyes)

| Diagnosis | *n* | Anatomical | | Visual | | Visual acuity ≥1/50 | |
|---|---|---|---|---|---|---|---|
| | | 6 | 24 | 6 | 24 | 6 | 24 |
| All diagnoses | 483 | 76 | 70 | 65 | 56 | 68 | 61 |
| ≥ 6 mos. follow-up | 400 | 78 | 72 | 71 | 61 | 72 | 65 |
| PVR, total | 226 | 72 | 63 | 67 | 55 | 65 | 60 |
| without perforating injury | 181 | 74 | 68 | 67 | 58 | 69 | 63 |
| with perforating injury | 45 | 65 | 44 | 68 | 42 | 50 | 46 |
| with giant tears | 20 | 59 | 52 | 54 | 29 | 44 | 44 |
| with posterior holes | 23 | 74 | 67 | 60 | 49 | 61 | 61 |
| PVR, uncomplicated | 144 | 75 | 68 | 71 | 62 | 72 | 65 |
| Stage C | 42 | 78 | 74 | 59 | 52 | 81 | 66 |
| Stage C1 | 8 | 88 | 88 | 75 | 75 | 88 | 88 |
| Stage C2 | 22 | 81 | 73 | 67 | 60 | 86 | 64 |
| Stage C3 | 12 | 65 | 65 | 33 | 22 | 67 | 55 |
| Stage D | 102 | 74 | 66 | 76 | 66 | 69 | 64 |
| Stage D1 | 27 | 89 | 89 | 85 | 81 | 78 | 78 |
| Stage D2 | 58 | 66 | 55 | 70 | 58 | 65 | 59 |
| Stage D3 | 17 | 75 | 62 | 82 | 64 | 65 | 55 |
| Giant tears, total | 70 | 84 | 82 | 71 | 62 | 73 | 68 |
| uncomplicated | 45 | 93 | 93 | 75 | 72 | 82 | 76 |
| Posterior holes, total | 71 | 83 | 77 | 72 | 62 | 75 | 72 |
| uncomplicated | 47 | 89 | 83 | 79 | 70 | 83 | 79 |
| MH, uncomplicated | 21 | 95 | 95 | 76 | 69 | 90 | 82 |
| PDR,total | 136 | 73 | 68 | 59 | 51 | 65 | 56 |
| with detachment | 124 | 71 | 67 | 55 | 49 | 63 | 56 |
| without detachment | 12 | 83 | 83 | 92 | 70 | 83 | 63 |
| Perforating injury, total | 61 | 69 | 54 | 68 | 49 | 55 | 53 |
| Other diagnoses | 13 | 51 | 51 | 15 | 15 | 30 | 30 |

PVR, proliferative vitreoretinopathy; MH, macular hole; PDR, proliferative diabetic retinopathy

[1]Values constitute cumulative proportions

### 3.1.1 Anatomic Success

At the last follow-up examination, after 21.7 months on average, the retina was completely attached in 350 of 483 eyes (72.5%; Table 5).

By life table analysis anatomic success after 6 months had been achieved in 76% of the eyes. The anatomic success rate thereafter showed a slightly decreasing tendency, which stabilized at about 70% after 2 years and which could mainly be attributed to redetachment through reproliferation.

The development of the anatomic success rates over time for all eyes and for eyes with the most important well-defined clinical pictures is displayed in Fig. 11. These subgroups add up to 433 eyes out of a whole sample of 483 eyes, but they are characterized by not having additional complicating factors, rather only those problems that were specific to their diagnosis. They correspond largely to the subgroups in Tables 5 and 6 marked "uncomplicated".

Of 144 eyes, 103 (71.5%) with *PVR* (uncomplicated) were operated on successfully. By life table analysis this was a success rate of 75% after 6 months and 68% after 24 months (early group: 67% and 57%, respectively; late group: 80% and 76%, respectively).The differences between early and late group already existed at the time of discharge (92% success in

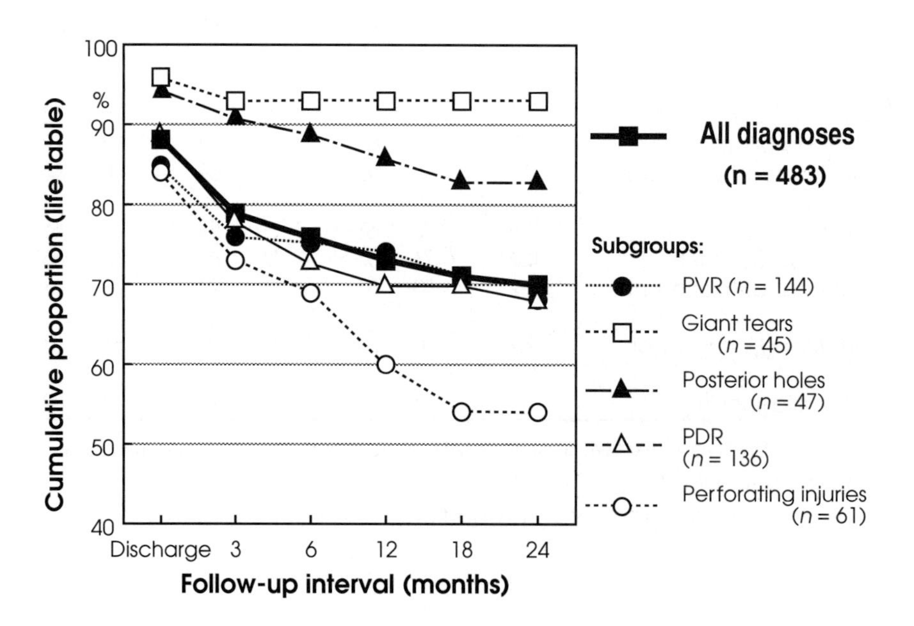


**Fig. 11.** Anatomic success after silicone oil surgery for the total cohort and those eyes with the most important well-defined clinical pictures (life table analysis)

the late group and 73% in the early group). After discharge the rate of failure through redetachment amounted to 16% for the following 2 years for each group. A detailed analysis of the late group (sufficient data were available only there) showed that 7 of 19 failures developed intraoperatively or immediately postoperatively. The cause of failure in the remaining 12 eyes was late reproliferation. In another 42 eyes, later successfully cured, one or several revision operations had to be performed because of reproliferation with redetachment. Thus, 54 out of 82 primarily successfully operated on eyes (66%) developed renewed retinal detachment through reproliferation. In 42 of these 54 redetachments, (78%) we were able to reattach the retina successfully, and 4 of the 12 eyes with uncured redetachment still had an attached macula with ambulatory vision and the possibility of further revisions. Only 8 of the 82 initially successfully operated on eyes (10%) became inoperable due to reproliferation.

The success rates for 6 and 12 months by life table analysis have been broken down for the different stages of PVR in Fig. 12. There is no clear correlation between stage of PVR and success rate.

*Giant tears* without PVR had an above-average anatomical success rate of 93%, both absolutely and by life table analysis. Only 3 of the 45 un-

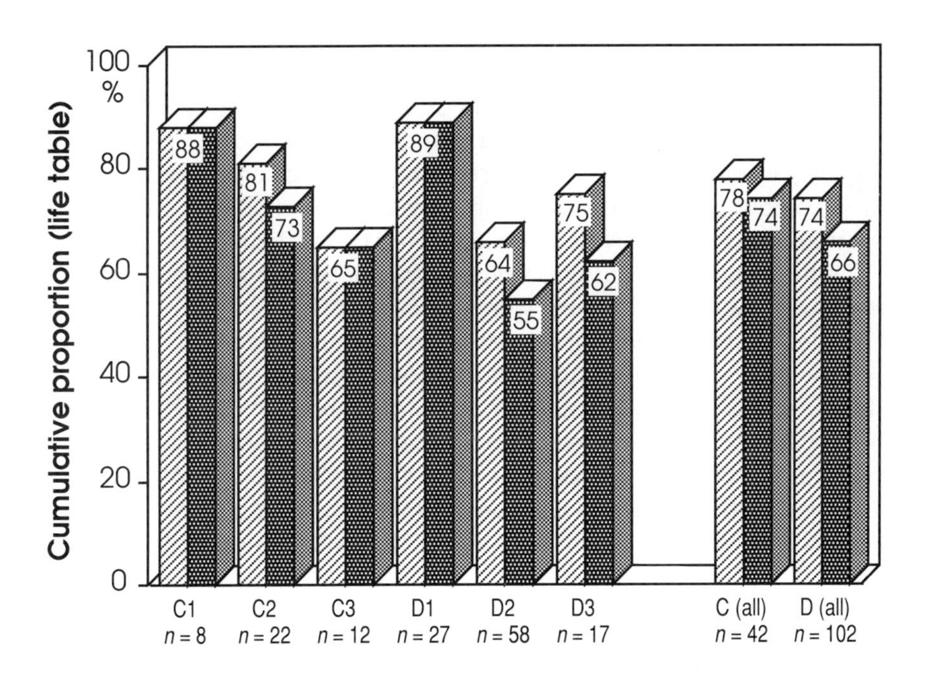


**Fig. 12.** Cumulative anatomic success rates in the various stages of PVR after 6 (▨) and 24 (▩) months

complicated giant tears were failures, all 3 had a size of about 180°. We equally succeeded in attaching both smaller and larger giant tears. A correlation between success rate and giant tear size could not be established and there was no difference between early and late groups.Two of the three failures had already ocurred intraoperatively because of massive choroidal hemorrhage. The third failure was a patient with an iatrogenic giant tear caused by an attempted cryoextraction of a lens nucleus lost during phakoemulsification. This was a heavily traumatized eye with vitreous hemorrhage which ended in disaster as a result of massive inflammation and intraocular proliferation. It is included with the "uncomplicated" giant tears as the giant tear was less than 24 h old and no clear evidence of PVR existed at that time.

In a total of 17 of the 42 successfully operated on giant tears at least one surgical revision was necessary. In six eyes this consisted in the removal of a thin preretinal membrane without retinal traction at the time of silicone oil removal. An additional four eyes developed a redetachment due to a clinically visible membrane that caused traction. In ten eyes revision was necessary to treat fresh retinal tears that had developed in areas outside the original giant tear. Membranes in the sense of a PVR were not found in the process. In summary we have seen membrane formation in 10 of 42 (24%) successfully operated on giant tears.

Of the 47 *posterior holes*, 7 were failures. This was a total success rate of 85.1% (83% after 2 years by life table analysis). As with the giant tears, no difference between the early and late groups was found. The results of surgery for macular holes were even better: there was only 1 failure among 21 uncomplicated macular holes. This was an eye with a very deep posterior staphyloma, in which the retina could not be reattached.

Of the remaining six failures with posterior holes one eye with subretinal silicone oil instillation resulted in intraoperative disaster; in the remaining five eyes membrane formation was responsible for the failure.

Among the 40 successfully operated on eyes we observed only 1 instance of membrane formation necessitating revision; 5 additional revision operations were necessary because of insufficient silicone oil filling and thus incomplete tamponade of the defects. No membranes were identified in the process. Consequently, membrane formation in the sense of a PVR occurred in 5 of the 47 eyes (11%) with posterior holes without PVR.

In 86 of 124 diabetics with *PDR* and traction detachment (69.4%), anatomic success was achieved by the last follow-up. By life table statistics the success rate was 71% after 6 months and 67% after 24 months.

Since the number of eyes in the early and late groups differed greatly, these two groups were not comparable.

In the subgroup of 12 diabetics who originally had no detachment and received silicone oil only for the purpose of hemostasis, late proliferation and thus failure developed in two eyes. The life table rates were 83% for both 6 and 24 months.

The worst success rates by far were found in eyes with *perforating injuries*. The retina was attached at the last follow-up examination in only 37 of 61 operated on eyes (60.7%), and the rate of late redetachments was particularly high. Whereas after 6 months 69% of the retinas were still attached, as calculated by life table analysis, this value deteriorated to 54% after 2 years. In the late group, however, the 2 year success rate was improved upon: 61% as compared to 46% in the early group.

As the group of other diagnoses was small and heterogeneous, statistical analyses were pointless. Only in 7 of the 13 eyes could a reattachment of the retina be achieved. Failures were noted in three patients, one with uveitis, one with a massive subretinal hemorrhage, and one with multiple retinal defects. Three more failures had to be attributed to acute retinal necrosis. Our experience with this disease has previously been published (Lucke et al. 1988).

### 3.1.2 Visual Success

The preoperative visual acuities and those at the time of the last follow-up examination are shown in Fig. 13.

It can easily be seen that in most eyes a visual improvement from counting fingers or light perception to 1/50 or 0.1 could be achieved. In some instances larger improvements to reading vision and even 1.0 (one patient) took place. Patients who had good visual acuity preoperatively but no ambulatory vision at the end of the follow-up period were very rare. The great majority of eyes with poor functional results in the end already had poor visual acuities preoperatively. Visual success rates by life table analysis are shown in Fig. 14 for all eyes and for the indication groups defined above.

Visual success rates were lower than anatomic ones. There was a difference of 11% at 6 months and of 14% at 24 months between the two success rates. These differences represent a group of eyes that had surgical successes, but did not achieve a recognizable improvement in visual acuity.

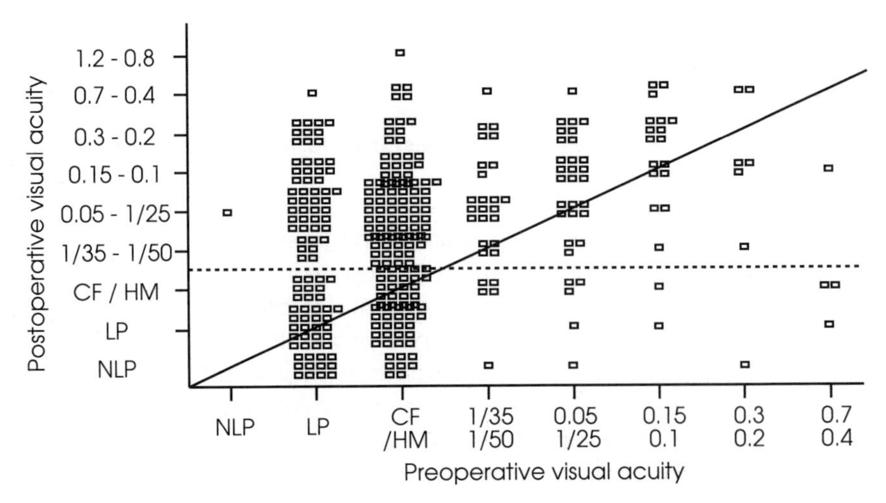


**Fig. 13.** Visual acuity preoperatively and at the last follow-up examination ($n$ = 483). The *dots* above the *diagonal* represent eyes with a postoperative visual acuity that improved over the preoperative one. This was true of 283 of the 483 eyes (58.6%). *Dots* above the *horizontal* line represent eyes that had ambulatory vision at the last examination. *CF,* counting fingers, *HM,* hand movement, *LP,* light perception, *NLP,* no light perception

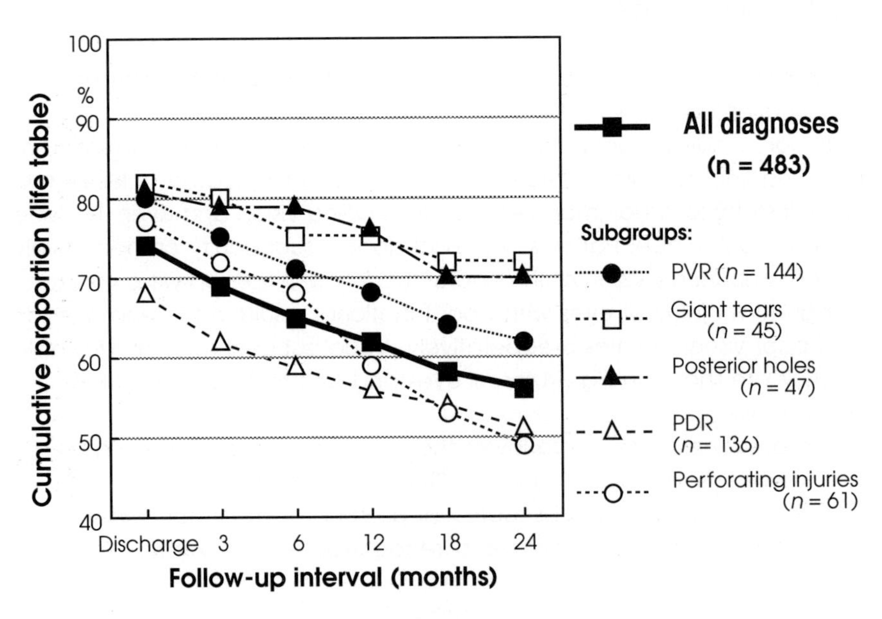


**Fig. 14.** Visual success after silicone oil surgery for the total cohort and those eyes with the most important well-defined clinical pictures (life table analysis)

### 3.1.3 Preservation of Ambulatory Vision

At the time of the last follow-up examination 313 of 483 patients (64.8%) still had an ambulatory visual acuity of 1/50 or better after an average 21.7 months. Life table values for this criterion were 68% at 6 months and 61% at 24 months. The difference relative to anatomic success was 8% after 6 months and 9% after 24 months. The results by life table statistics are shown in Fig. 15 for all eyes and the defined indication groups.

In all indication groups the percentage of eyes with preserved ambulatory vision was below that for anatomic success. Possible reasons are dealt with in Sect. 3.1.4. As was expected considering the anatomic results, ambulatory vision could be best preserved in eyes with posterior holes and giant tears and least in perforating injuries and diabetics. By this success criterion, the differences between the early and late groups were considerably higher than by anatomic success rates. Whereas the difference between ambulatory vision and anatomic success at 6 and 24 months was 15% and 13%, respectively, in the early group, this difference decreased to 4% and 6% in the late group.

A visual acuity of 1/50 or better at the last follow-up examination was

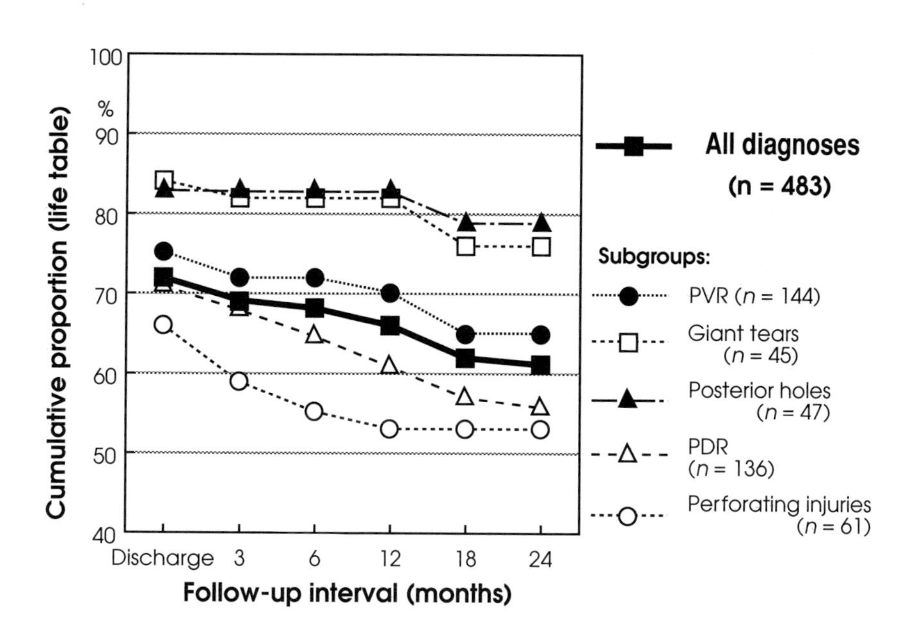


**Fig. 15.** Preservation of ambulatory vision (visual acuity ≥1/50) for the total cohort and those eyes with the most important well-defined clinical pictures (life table analysis)

achieved in 69.4% of eyes with *uncomplicated PVR*. The respective life table rates were 72% after 6 months and 65% after 2 years. There were considerable differences between early and late groups. The life table rates for the early group were 56% after 6 months and 49% after 24 months, whereas the comparative values in the late group were 82% and 74%, respectively.

The difference was even greater with *giant tears*. Whereas 68% of the uncomplicated giant tears in the early group had ambulatory vision after 2 years, this increased to 93% in the late group.

Even though in eyes with *posterior holes* the defect is in the macular area, 83% of the eyes achieved a visual acuity of 1/50 or better after 6 months and 79% after 2 years. There was no difference between the early and the late group.

The functional results in *diabetics* were relatively poor. By life table analysis, ambulatory vision was achieved in 65% of the eyes after 6 months, but this value deteriorated to 56% after 24 months. These constituted the highest visual losses between the 6th and the 24th month (9%). The difference relative to the anatomic success rate (12% at 2 years) was relatively large as well.

Corresponding with the percentage of anatomic successes, the percentage of eyes with ambulatory vision in the group of *perforating injuries* was the lowest of all indications: 55% after 6 months and 53% after 2 years by life table analysis. The rate of loss between 6 and 24 months was relatively low (2%); there was, however, a high rate of loss between discharge and the 6 month interval (11%).

### 3.1.4 Poor Visual Acuity in Spite of Attached Retina

The figures above show that there is a certain percentage of eyes which did not achieve satisfactory visual function in spite of an attached retina. Figure 16 shows the proportion of eyes with ambulatory vision from those with attached retinas at the end of follow-up.

In all 66 eyes had no ambulatory vision at the last examination in spite of attached retinas, i.e., 14% of the the whole sample and 19% of the patients successfully operated on. We should like to analyze this cohort further since such functional failures constituted a considerable proportion of the successfully operated on patients, and the causes of such functional losses are of great importance for the assessment of the safety of silicone oil.

Virtually all indication groups were involved, although to a different degree. The causes of these losses of visual acuity were analyzed in detail and the results are summarized in Table 7.

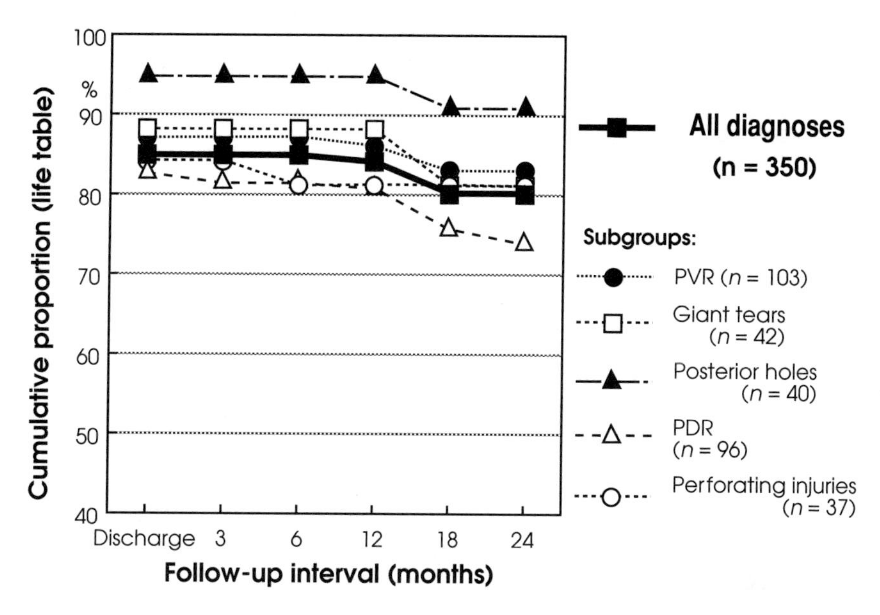


**Fig. 16.** Preservation of ambulatory vision in eyes with attached retinas for the total cohort and those eyes with the most important well-defined clinical pictures (life table analysis)

The most frequent causes were retinal or optic nerve atrophies. Usually factors could easily be identified which could be regarded as probable causes from a clinical point of view after elimination of other possibilities. Nonetheless there is no final proof for these interpretations and the distribution in Table 7 may very well not be free of prejudice.

Diabetic and other vasculopathies were regarded as probable causes of retinal atrophy in 19 eyes. Particularly in diabetic eyes, retinal atrophy progressed in spite of retinal reattachment and sometimes led to loss of function. In three patients the retinal detachment had existed for more than 6 months, and function did not regenerate in spite of good reattachment. In six patients hypotony and phthisis developed, twice after perforating injury, twice (with PVR) after multiple surgical trauma, and twice (giant tears) due to a string syndrome developing postoperatively.

In one patient an endophthalmitis had preceded, leaving the retina without function; in one patient with iatrogenic perforation of the eye during retrobulbar anesthesia, retinal atrophy could be attributed to toxic retinal damage by the injected anesthetic agent, and in four patients the retina did not recover in spite of reattachment after massive choroidal or subretinal hemorrhage.

**Table 7.** Causes for poor visual acuity in spite of attached retina

| Cause | *n* |
|---|---|
| Retinal or optic nerve atrophy | |
| Diabetic vasculopathy | 15 |
| Other vasculopathies[1] | 4 |
| Old detachment | 3 |
| Hypotony/phthisis | 6 |
| Endophthalmitis | 1 |
| Toxic retinal damage | 1 |
| Severe choroidal detachment, subretinal hemorrhage | 4 |
| Keratopathy | 9 |
| Cataract | 7 |
| Macular pucker | 1 |
| Macular scar | 2 |
| No clear cause identifiable | 13[2] |
| Total | 66 |

[1]Including acute retinal necrosis, uveitis, and Eales.
[2]Including 9 with a follow-up less than 3 months.

In nine patients poor visual acuity was attributed to a keratopathy; eight of those were in the early group, in which keratopathies were much more frequent than later on (see below).

In one patient a distinct macular pucker and in two other patients macular scars were responsible for poor visual acuity.

In 13 patients the cause of poor visual acuity could not be determined clinically; however, in 9 of them the follow-up was less than 3 months. The remaining four belonged to the early group, and the cause of poor visual acuity could not be determined any more.

We did not find any clinical clues suggestive of toxic damage by the silicone oil itself.

## 3.1.5 Development of Visual Acuity

### 3.1.5.1 Average Visual Acuity

To examine the question whether any retinotoxic effect could possibly be detected in the development of visual acuity, we studied the changes in average visual performance. We eliminated factors that might influence visual acuity in ways other than by possible toxicity and therefore selected from the whole cohort those eyes that had attached retinas during the entire follow-up period and who developed neither raised intraocular pressures nor keratopathies: 231 eyes met these criteria. An average visual acuity was calculated for each follow-up interval and each patient cohort. The results are shown in Fig. 17.

Whereas preoperatively the average visual acuity roughly amounted to hand movement, it increased to about 0.05-0.1 after 6 months in the 231 eyes, decreased slightly again after 12 months, and reached a maximum value after 2 years. Although the decrease after 12 months was within the range of statistical error, the interrupted lines in the graph show the probable cause. Here the average visual performances were analyzed in two subgroups of 74 eyes each. The eyes in one group were already aphakic preoperatively or the lens had been removed in the initial operation so that the postoperative visual acuity was at no time influenced by the development of a cataract. The second group was phakic during the whole time of observation including the last follow-up examination and therefore virtually all eyes had a cataract in the end. The comparison of the curves shows clearly the parallel development of visual acuity up to the 6 month interval; the curves thereafter diverge due to the development of cataract. Consistent with clinical experience, cataract caused a significant deterioration of visual acuity usually between the 6th and the 12th

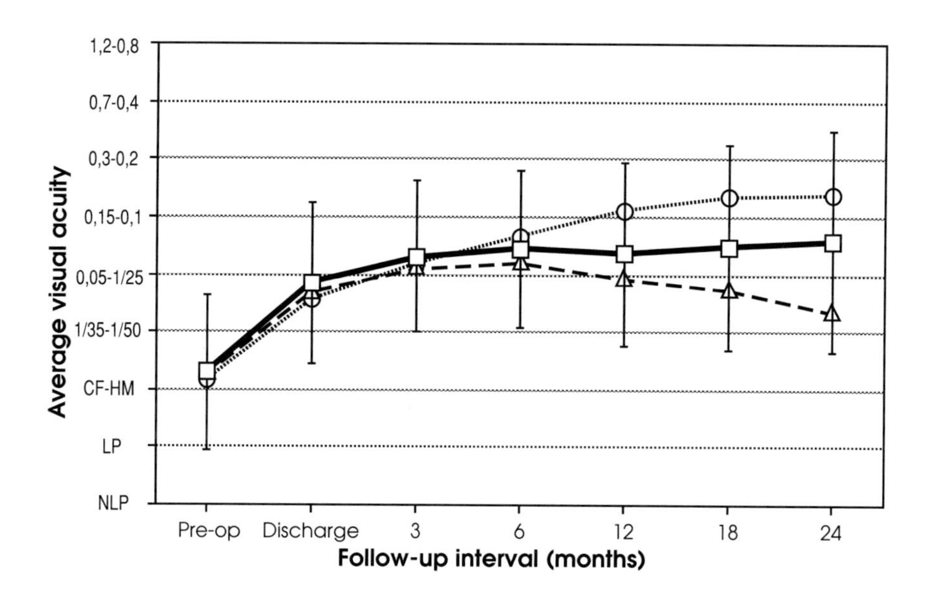


**Fig. 17.** Development of visual acuity in eyes with attached retinas (without glaucoma or keratopathy). —□— All eyes ($n$ = 231); ···○··· Eyes already aphakic preoperatively ($n$ = 74); – –△– – Eyes, still phakic at the end of follow-up ($n$ = 74). The *error bars* (1 standard deviation) are shown for the large cohort only; *CF*, counting fingers; *HM*, hand movement; *LP*, light perception; *NLP*, no light perception

month. If the cataract factor is eliminated, no dip in the curve, which could be interpreted as a possible clue to retinal toxicity, can be seen. On the contrary, the average visual acuity still continues to improve up to the 18th month and even slightly thereafter to a value of about 0.15-0.2.

#### 3.1.5.2 Average Visual Acuity and Silicone Oil Removal

A further way of examining possible toxic effects of silicone oil consists of comparing retinal function in eyes from which the silicone oil was removed with that in those eyes in which the silicone oil was left in for a long time period. Here too, only eyes that had an attached retina and showed neither glaucoma nor keratopathy should be considered. Furthermore, as the analysis above has shown, they should have been aphakic at least at the last follow-up examination to eliminate the effect of cataract formation if possible. A total of 152 eyes met these criteria. A restriction to eyes that had been aphakic throughout would have resulted in too small a sample. The silicone oil had been removed from 91 of the 152 eyes at the time of the last follow-up examination. These eyes thus represented a group in which the proportion filled with silicone oil decreased with time until the oil had been removed in practically all eyes after 24 months at the latest.

The control group of 61 eyes had silicone oil in the eye during the whole time of observation. The curves of the development of visual acuity in these two cohorts are shown in Fig. 18.

In both groups a temporary dip in average visual acuity around the 12th month, probably caused by cataract, is found again as in Fig. 17. The eyes from which the silicone oil was removed showed a much better development of visual acuity than those in which we left the oil in situ. It is, however, surprising that the difference between the two curves was already clearly established at 3 months, at a time when the great majority of the eyes in the removal group still had the oil in the eye (the timing of silicone oil removal is discussed on p. 56). Consequently, the differences in visual performance between the two cohorts could hardly be attributed to a toxic effect of silicone oil. More likely, that those eyes in which we left the oil in situ represent a selection with a more complicated pathology that were probably not capable of better visual performance for reasons of their disease. Continuing this kind of analysis beyond 24 months is pointless in our sample, since the number of patients with oil still in situ that long after initial surgery becomes too small to be analyzed with any significance.

On the basis of the development of average visual acuity, a retinotoxic effect of silicone oil can therefore not be established. Although this does not mean that there might not be one, factors such as cataract, keratopathy, and intrinsic retinal factors related to the disease itself are probably considerably more significant influences on visual performance.

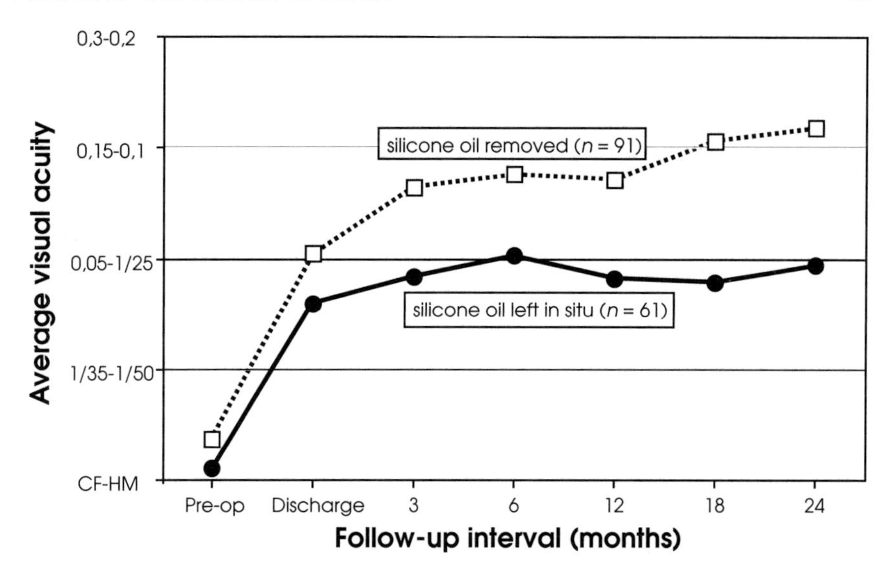


**Fig. 18.** Average visual performance in relation to silicone oil removal (eyes with attached retinas, without glaucoma or keratopathy, aphakic at the last follow-up examination). CF, counting fingers; HM, hand movements

## 3.2 Special Problems

### 3.2.1 Number of Operations

As mentioned before (p. 16), 49% of the eyes had been operated on once or several times previous to silicone oil surgery. Counting from the first silicone oil operation, a total of 948 operations on 483 eyes were performed. This amounts to 1.96 operations per eye on average.

On the 350 successes 724 operations in all were performed (2.06 per eye) as compared to 224 operations performed on the 133 failures (1.68 per eye). The difference is explained by the fact that in only 17 of the failures was the silicone oil removed for good, in contrast to 168 of the 350 successes (48%). It cannot be deduced from the figures that an aggressive surgical strategy is partly responsible for anatomic success.

Taking into account that in 182 of the successes the oil was still in situ and still had to be removed, it can be calculated that *at least* 906 operations, i.e., 2.6 operations per eye on average, were needed to achieve final anatomic success. This figure differs only insignificantly in the various indication groups (PVR, 2.79; giant tears:, 2.79; posterior holes, 2.32; diabetics, 2.40; perforating injuries, 2.49).

If we include the silicone oil removals that were still pending, and assume that these would not lead to redetachment, anatomic success was achieved with a minimum of two operations in 223 of the 350 successes (64%). A further 76 eyes (22%) needed an additional revision operation, while in the remaining 51 (15%) four or more surgical procedures proved necessary.

These figures are indicative of the fact that this surgical method is more suitable for particularly motivated patients, i.e. mainly those with one eye or bilateral involvement. Although we do use it frequently in patients with a good contralateral eye, the fact that several operations will be needed must be clearly explained in the preoperative talk with the patient. This is an "extreme" form of surgery not only in its technique, but also in the expense involved.

### 3.2.2 Results After Silicone Oil Removal

The fate of all 483 eyes with regard to the removal of silicone oil is summarized in Fig. 19 in the form of a flowchart.

Some 121 eyes were primary failures; we did not remove the silicone oil from most of these as they usually tolerate silicone oil quite well for a long time. At the last follow-up examination 116 failures still had oil in the eye; 11 of them, however, were later enucleated.

In 169 of the 362 primary successes we left the silicone oil in because it seemed not to be an appropriate time for silicone oil removal, removal was regarded as too risky, or the patients had reservations about removal. There were 13 eyes in which the oil had to be reinjected after an attempted removal. These have to be added to the 169; thus 182 of the 483 eyes with attached retinas still had silicone oil in situ at the last examination.

There were 193 eyes from which we tried to remove the silicone oil that represent a special group. In 30 of these 193 silicone oil removals with attached retinas (15%), problems developed postoperatively through redetachment (27 times,14%), recurrent bleeding with diabetes (once), or hypotony (twice). The frequency of silicone oil removals in the individual indication groups is listed in Table 8.

The proportions of attempted silicone oil removals vary widely in the various indication groups. We removed the oil in 33 of 42 giant tears (79%), for example, but only in 36 of 98 diabetics (37%). The rates of redetachments, e.g.,18% in patients with giant tears and 8% in diabetics, differed likewise. Possible explanations will be dealt with in Chap. 4.

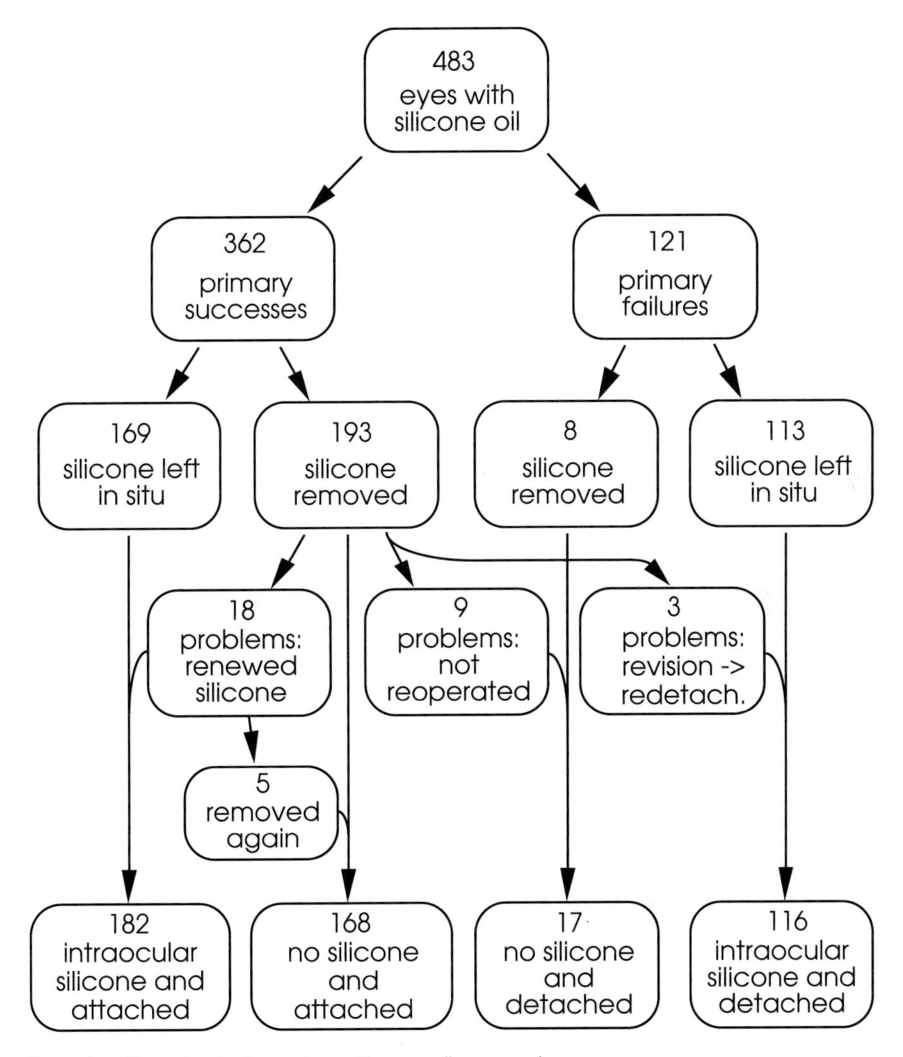


**Fig. 19.** Flowchart of results of silicone oil removal

We revised 18 of the 27 eyes with redetachment by reinjecting silicone oil and did likewise in the patient with recurrent bleeding and the two patients with hypotony. In all but three eyes this led to the desired success. In five of the eyes the oil was later removed again (Fig. 19). No revision was attempted in nine eyes either because the situation was hopeless or because the patient refused it. Accordingly, 12 of the 193 attempted silicone oil removals (6.2%) ended with a redetachment; in 93.8% the retina was attached at the last follow-up examination.

**Table 8.** Problems after silicone oil removal in cases with attached retina

| | *n* | % | Redetachment (%) | | Hemorrhage | Hypotony |
|---|---|---|---|---|---|---|
| All eyes | 193/362 | 53 | 27/193 | 14 | 1/193 | 2/193 |
| Early group | 96/134 | 72 | 15/96 | 16 | 1/96 | 2/96 |
| Late group | 97/228 | 43 | 12/97 | 12 | | |
| PVR, no injury | 69/131 | 53 | 10/69 | 14 | | 2/69 |
| Giant tears | 33/42 | 79 | 6/33 | 18 | | |
| Posterior holes | 29/42 | 69 | 2/29 | 7 | | |
| Diabetes | 36/98 | 37 | 3/36 | 8 | 1/36 | |
| Perforating Injury | 23/40 | 58 | 4/23 | 17 | | |
| Others | 3/13 | 23 | 2/3 | 67 | | |

### 3.2.3 Timing of Silicone Oil Removal

To better define when and why we removed the silicone oil, the main group of patients with successful silicone oil removals with attached retinas was examined more closely. In these 168 eyes, silicone oil removal was performed after 12.2 months on average. The timing was, however, extremely variable and ranged from 3 weeks to 64 months after the initial operation. The distribution is shown in Fig. 20.

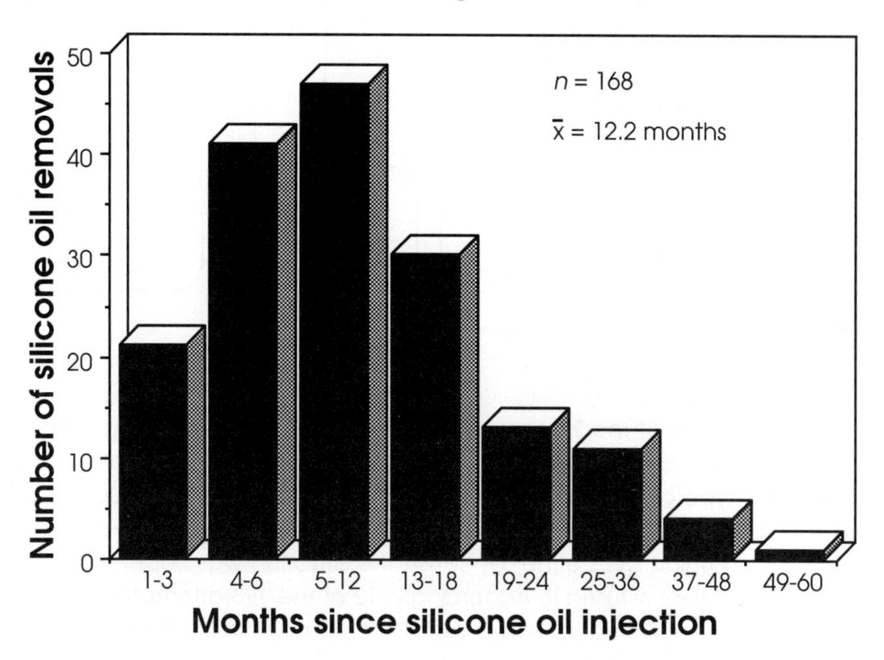


**Fig. 20.** Timing of silicone oil removal in eyes with attached retinas

The main reason for deciding to remove the silicone oil was, in most cases, the impression that the oil was no longer needed for tamponade. This situation existed when the retina was stable, attached, and without remnants of proliferation. There were additional factors involved in the decision such as complications that had already developed (e.g., glaucoma, keratopathy, and cataract reducing visual acuity), danger of late complications, and problems in the logistics of further postoperative care.

Although for each patient the exact motive for silicone oil removal can no longer be reconstructed, we shall nevertheless try to show the resulting trends based on the available data.

#### 3.2.3.1 Lens Extraction

A frequent motive for early removal of silicone oil was, in the beginning, the thought of protecting the lens against cataract formation. Accordingly, the lens was retained in 25 of 58 silicone oil removals in phakic eyes (43%) in the early group, while in 33 eyes (47%) the lens was removed at the same time (another 38 eyes were already aphakic at the time of silicone oil removal). When only two of the 25 preserved lenses remained permanently clear, however, the strategy was changed so that in the late group, examined here in greater detail, 57 of 64 silicone oil removals in phakic eyes (89%) were carried out simultaneously with lens extraction. This usually happened when the cataract affected visual acuity significantly. In the late group the oil was removed early in order to save the lens if possible in only four patients (twice successfully so far). In three patients a cloudy lens was temporarily retained on purpose in order to be able to perform an extracapsular cataract extraction with lens implantation a few weeks later.

#### 3.2.3.2 Aphakic eyes

In the late group 33 eyes were already aphakic at the time of silicone oil removal. In these eyes keratopathy (three eyes) and glaucoma (seven eyes) had at least a share in the decision to remove the silicone oil. In the remaining eyes motives such as prevention of such complications and logistic considerations were the more pertinent ones.

#### 3.2.3.3 Reasons for Retention of Silicone Oil

In a great number of patients in the late group silicone oil removal was still pending. In 32 eyes, the oil had already remained in place for more than 18 months,. These patients had a completely attached retina and satisfactory visual function (≥1/50). Nonetheless the question arises why the oil was not removed.

Six of these eye were phakic, but the cataract was not so marked that lens and silicone oil removal were necessary; thus removal was pending as well. In two patients a revision of the retina was necessary at the time of lens extraction which had not been all that long ago. Two eyes suffered from hypotony and the oil was left in situ as prophylaxis against shrinkage. In one patient silicone oil removal was planned for the near future. In the remaining patients, there was a lack of certainty whether the retina was already securely attached and a lack of motivation on the part of the patients to have a potentially risky operation performed when function is satisfactory and conditions are stable. After all, 12 of the 21 patients concerned had already undergone one or several revision procedures, and in four eyes the silicone oil had already been removed once and a redetachment had developed. Thus reservations towards silicone oil removal were understandable, particularly since proof of silicone oil toxicity is outstanding.

There were, however, some patients who were not being followed-up intensively enough for logistic reasons and in whom the oil remained in the eye for an unnecessarily long time. In some respects this can be seen as a disadvantage of silicone oil surgery.

## 3.3 Complications

In surgery of such complexity complications cannot be avoided. The difficulty is to distinguish effectively between complications attributable to the basic disease, the vitreoretinal operation, the direct retinal surgery, or the silicone oil itself. An analysis of complications can best be divided into problems developing intraoperatively and those developing postoperatively.

### 3.3.1 Intraoperative Complications

Intraoperative complications can, on the one hand, be the result of standard vitreoretinal procedures that are a part of such surgery. They have already been described at length in the literature (Machemer and Aaberg 1981, Michels 1981, Schepens 1983, Charles 1981) and need not be further analyzed here.

Of the special complications which may, on the other hand, arise because of the use of silicone oil or because of the extreme retinal surgery, the *prolapse of silicone oil under the retina*, often associated with *retinal rupture*, is probably the most important. Altogether this complication arose 13 times in our series: 12 times during the first 100 operations but only once afterwards. In the latter it was, however, possible to attach the retina successfully after generous retinectomy; in the former this complication led to failure. This complication arises when silicone oil is injected before the retina is free of traction, and must be regarded as an avoidable complication.

In five operations *silicone oil* went past the lens *into the anterior chamber* intraoperatively, twice in the early group, and three times in the late group. In one operation it happened when we attempted to reposition an intraocular lens in an eye already filled with silicone oil, and once it was caused by the infusion cannula being tilted too far forward so that during silicone oil injection the oil was pressed through the zonula into the anterior chamber. In the other three operations too vehement manipulation of the eye caused the silicone oil to be pressed forward. In one of these five eyes we immediately performed a lensectomy. In another one the silicone bubble was so small that it could be left in the anterior chamber and in the remaining 3 cases we removed the silicone oil from the anterior chamber using Healon in a technique described by Kirkby and Gregor (1987).

In one eye we inadvertently injected a small amount of *silicone oil into the choroid* due to a poorly positioned infusion cannula. The mistake was noticed quickly and the cannula repositioned. The incident was without consequences; the retina remained attached, and a persisting choroidal detachment was not seen.

The formation of *iatrogenic retinal holes* during preretinal membrane peeling must be counted among the complications of direct retinal surgery. It is a frequent occurrence and a decisive indication for the use of silicone oil as already discussed above.

Larger retinectomies may lead to massive *hemorrhages* sometimes hard to control. In cases of PVR with massive retinal shortening a big circumferential retinectomy may cause slipping or clumping of the retina at the posterior pole or even *tulip formation* which can be very difficult to manage. In recent years these complications have been observed in rare instances. We have not analyzed them in detail.

## 3.3.2 Postoperative Complications

In the analysis of postoperative complications we should also like to restrict ourselves to those which we think could be attributed particularly to extreme vitreoretinal surgery and to those eyes in which the retina was attached at the end of the observation period. The natural course of serious retinal detachments without surgery includes a great number of complications such as cataract, glaucoma, hypotony, phthisis, and band keratopathy, so that an analysis of complications in eyes with anatomic failure cannot yield much pertinent information. With regard to complications, it is more important, of course, to find out whether an anatomic success was possibly thwarted by secondary complications. In the following we shall therefore limit our discussion to the complications in those 350 eyes in which we were able to reattach the retina successfully.

The most important postoperative complications were cataract, emulsification, glaucoma, rubeosis iridis, and keratopathy. Silicone oil prolapse and the problem of closed inferior iridectomies will be considered in the section on keratopathies (see Sect. 3.3.3.5). Endophthalmitis, scleral fistula formation, and hypotony were only rarely observed.

We will not separately investigate the problem of reproliferation, which, in fact, is often considered as a complication, but is actually a problem of the underlying disease. Moreover, it appears as an element in the statistics on anatomical failure, and it is discussed in detail on p. 85.

#### 3.3.2.1 Cataracts

As already mentioned above (p. 57), almost all phakic eyes developed a cataract in the course of events. In 29 eyes we removed the oil early to prevent cataract formation, but only 4 of them kept a clear lens for some time after initial surgery (12, 18, 52, and 55 months). In these the silicone oil was removed after 1, 3, 4, and 6 months; three of these four patients were diabetics.

In the final analysis we conclude that cataract formation is almost obligatory. In older patients this usually happens in the form of a nuclear sclerosis, which can later have a high water content. By contrast younger patients will more likely develop an opacification of the posterior lens cortex.

Cataract is a well-known complication after simple vitrectomies and has been reported in about 30% – 60% of patients depending on the length of follow-up (Michels 1984, de Bustros et al. 1988).

Corresponding to the rate of cataract development, the proportion of aphakic eyes increased continually during the observation period. Whereas 38% of all successfully operated on eyes were aphakic immediately after the initial operation, this proportion rose to 81% within 24 months by life table analysis (Fig. 21). In all indication groups the rate of increase was roughly parallel. As lenses were frequently involved in perforating injuries, the rate of aphakia in that indication group was considerably higher and reached 100% after 2 years. In the diabetics in whom we mostly preserved the lens primarily, the rate of aphakia was accordingly relatively low.

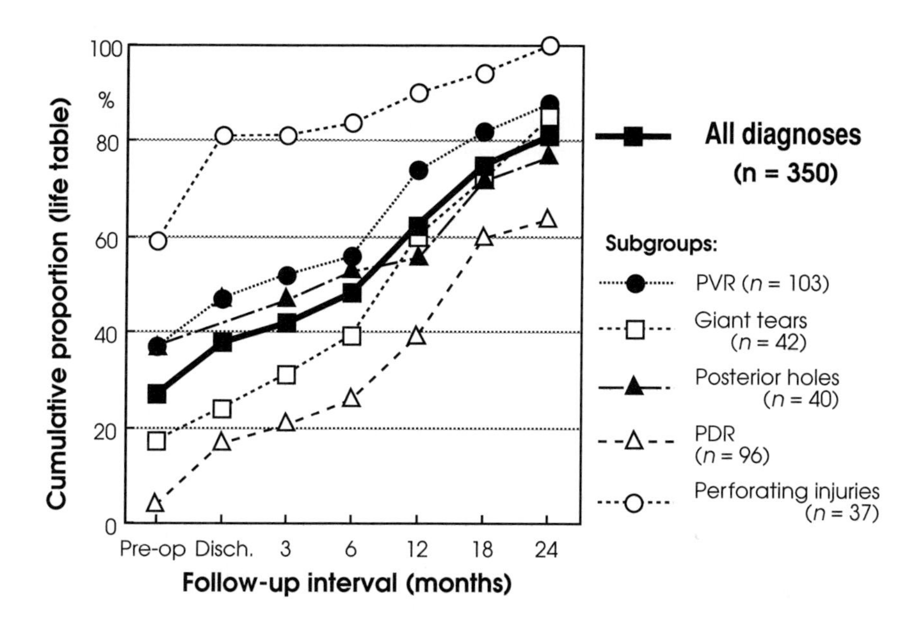


**Fig. 21.** Cumulative rate of aphakia in eyes with attached retinas for the total cohort and those eyes with the most important well-defined clinical pictures (life table analysis)

### 3.3.2.2 Emulsification

Droplet formation of silicone oil is usually referred to clinically as "emulsification". The mechanism leading to droplet formation is largely unknown. In theory such emulsification should be expected to always occur, at least in a mild form.

It is extremely difficult to record this emulsification statistically since thorough gonioscopy would reveal some degree of emulsification in the chamber angle at 12 o'clock and on the retina in the majority of eyes and furthermore since it has not yet been possible to satisfactorily quantify emulsification. Considering these difficulties, we can only state that we found a record of significant emulsification in the medical files of 24 patients (5%): 10 times in the early group (5.4%) who were operated on with an unpurified oil, 1000CS, and 14 times in the late group (4.7%) who received the purified oil OP5000. Although these figures suggest that there was no difference between the two oils, the clinical impression was that the extent of emulsification significantly decreased with introduction of the purified and more viscous silicone oil (see Color Plate 4, Figs. 3a +b). The discrepancy between statistics and clinical impression can perhaps be explained by the fact that awareness of the problem of emulsification has risen considerably in recent times and that we carried out regular examinations of the chamber angle for only a few years. It can be assumed that a considerable percentage of emulsifications were not recorded, particularly in the early group.

Emulsification is probably obligatory although for unexplained reasons it develops differently from patient to patient. It is very rarely clinically overt, particularly since the introduction of OP5000, and it is only of clinical importance if it leads to secondary glaucoma (pp. 63 and 65).

### 3.3.2.3 Glaucoma.

We have divided postoperatively occurring rises in intraocular pressure (secondary glaucoma) by clinical criteria into three groups:

1. *Pressure increases developing immediately postoperatively* could usually be attributed to inflammation or choroidal detachment. They sometimes persisted for up to 3 weeks and could be controlled in most instances by intensive local cortisone therapy. We have not considered them here in detail as they occur after all intraocular operations and are not specifically associated with silicone oil or extreme retinal surgery.

2. The second group was comprised of *temporary pressure* increases which developed or persisted postoperatively more than 3 weeks after surgery and normalized either spontaneously or as a result of treatment.

Such increases occurred in 25 eyes. Their probable causes are shown

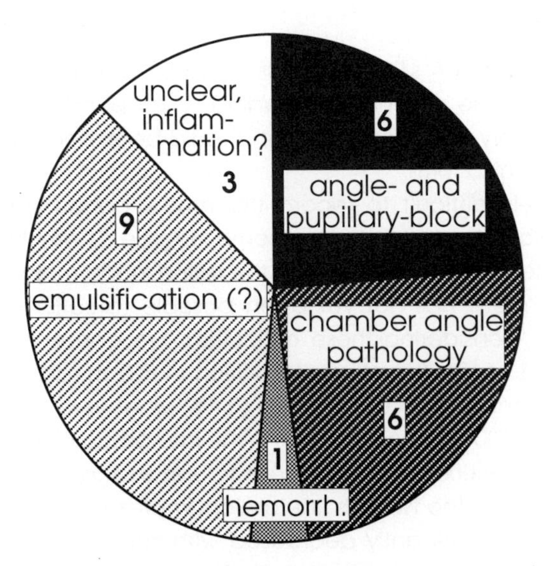


**Fig. 22.** Causes of temporary increases in intraocular pressure in eyes with attached retinas ($n = 25/350$)

graphically in Fig. 22.

In six eyes mechanical blocks were responsible: three times caused by silicone prolapse into the anterior chamber with a closed inferior iridectomy, once as a result of pupillary-block with a swelling lens, once due to occlusio pupillae, and once as a result of flattening of the anterior chamber and closure of the chamber angle with silicone oil pressing forward.

In another six eyes the chamber angle showed pathological changes: three times with complete aniridia after trauma, once with rubeosis iridis, and once with peripheral anterior synechiae. As such anatomic changes are generally not reversible, it must be assumed that the glaucoma problem was sometimes masked by a coexisting hypofunction of the ciliary body.

In one diabetic eye a temporary hemolytic glaucoma occurred after silicone oil removal due to secondary hemorrhage.

In nine eyes we suspected emulsification of the silicone oil as the cause of glaucoma. In five of them emulsification was clinically evident, three with an "inverse hypopion" (see Color Plate 4, Fig. 3a). In the remaining four eyes emulsification was rather mild; the intraocular pressure, however, spontaneously normalized after silicone oil removal.

In the remaining three eyes the cause of temporary rise in pressure was not clearly evident, but a temporary inflammatory state might have been causative.

About half of the temporary pressure increases therefore were probably caused by silicone oil in one way or another (angle- and pupillary blocks, emulsification), whereas the remaining increases were more likely attributable to causes specific to the underlying disease.

3. The third group, *persisting glaucoma* was comprised of those eyes that at the time of the last follow-up examination had an intraocular pressure of 25 mm Hg or higher, were dependent on glaucoma medication, or on which a cyclodiathermy, transscleral cw-YAG laser coagulation (Mehdorn et al. 1989), or cyclocryotherapy had been performed at any time after silicone oil surgery.

Before the silicone oil operation nine of the 350 eyes (3%) already had a glaucoma. By life table analysis the cumulative proportion of all eyes with persisting glaucoma rose to 15% after 2 years (Fig. 23).

The frequency of glaucoma in the various indication groups was rather variable. High rates of glaucoma were evident for patients with posterior holes and for diabetics. In the following we have supplemented the global statistical analysis by an individual analysis of the eyes concerned in order to try to obtain information on possible causes.

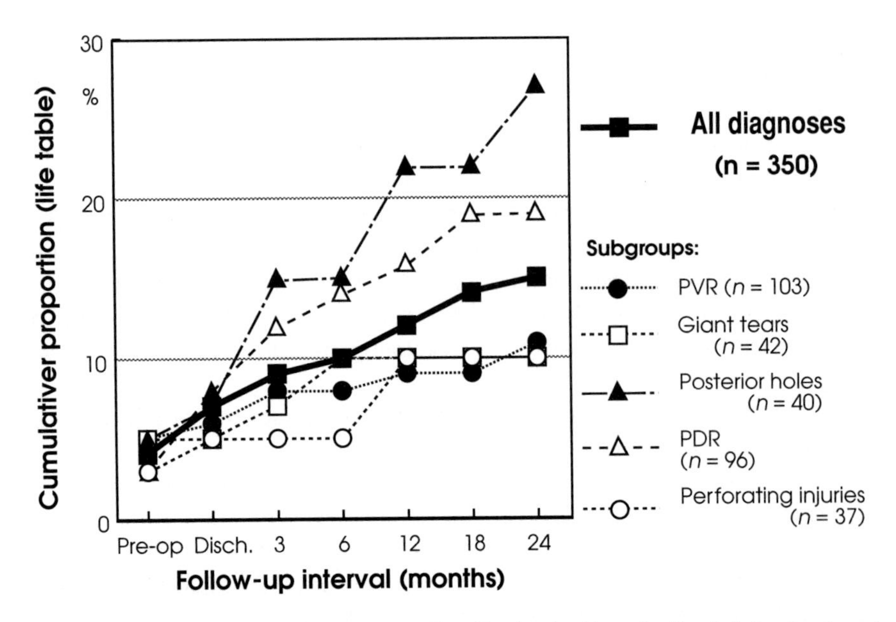


**Fig. 23.** Persisting glaucoma in eyes with attached retinas for the total cohort and those eyes with the most important well-defined clinical pictures (life table analysis)

There were 48 eyes in all that had a glaucoma at the last follow-up examination, nine of those, as mentioned, already had a glaucoma before the operation. Thus 39 eyes developed secondary glaucoma (39/350 = 11%).

Ten of these eyes had a *PVR* (glaucoma rate: 10/103 = 10%): In five of these eyes the chamber angle was completely or partially closed, in one due to the extension of the proliferative process to the anterior segment, in another through central retinal vein thrombosis and rubeosis iridis, and in three without clearly recognizable cause. One patient developed a secondary glaucoma due to marked emulsification, which at first did not improve after silicone oil removal because of persisting droplets. The remaining four patients were highly myopic. One also showed slight emulsification, which might have been a possible cause of the glaucoma; in another, with iatrogenic perforation (also with a high myopia), the chamber angle might have been damaged by a toxic effect (local anesthetic) or by massive secondary inflammation; and in a third, a mentally handicapped patient, damage of the chamber angle through contusion trauma, which was probably also responsible for the detachment, must be assumed as a possible cause.

Of 42 patients with uncomplicated *giant tears*, three (7%) developed a secondary glaucoma (one patient with high myopia already had a glaucoma preoperatively). High myopia was common to all three of them. In one patient it was associated with a Marfan's syndrome; another patient had a unilateral highly myopic, amblyopic eye (the other eye was normal), and another patient had meanwhile also developed a glaucoma in the eye not operated on.

Of 40 patients with *posterior holes*, seven (18%) had developed secondary glaucoma by the last follow-up examination. It is remarkable that again there was the same basic situation in all seven of these eyes: extremely high myopia with chorioatrophic scars at the posterior pole; slight emulsification; some inflammation; and slight, persisting, raised intraocular pressures, which were easily controlled by medication in all but one eye.

Altogether 16 of 96 eyes with *PDR* (17%) had a secondary glaucoma at the last follow-up examination. In seven of these a rubeosis iridis was documented.

Only two of 37 eyes with *perforating injury* (5%) developed a secondary glaucoma. One of them had increased pressure with slight emulsification only once, at the last follow-up examination. Silicone oil removal was planned for shortly thereafter. The other patient had increased pressure at discharge, but never appeared again so that speculations as to the cause are impossible.

Among the patients with *miscellaneous diagnoses* one developed a rubeosis with neovascular secondary glaucoma due to Eales' disease.

The probable main causes for the development of 39 cases of sec-

**Table 9.** Probable causes and possible identifiable risk factors for secondary glaucoma in cases with attached retina ($n = 39$)

| Cause or risk factor ($n$) | Total |
|---|---|
| Neovascular glaucoma | 18 |
| Diabetes (16) | |
| Eales' disease (1) | |
| Central retinal vein thrombosis (1) | |
| Peripheral anterior synechiae | 4 |
| Emulsification | 4 |
| High myopia (1) | |
| Uveitis (1) | |
| Glaucoma in the other eye as well (1) | |
| Inflammation | 4 |
| High myopia (1) | |
| No follow-up examination since discharge (2) | |
| Toxic ?, intraocular injection of local anesthetic (1) | |
| Causes unclear | 9 |
| Trauma (1) | |
| High myopia (7) | |

ondary glaucoma and the risk factors involved are summed up in Table 9.

Of the 39 instances of persisting secondary glaucoma 23 were satisfactorily controlled by medication alone at the last follow-up examination. This included all highly myopic eyes with posterior holes or giant tears. In six eyes the glaucoma was not treated because of poor visual function, and we were not able to reexamine another three patients since diagnosing the glaucoma and prescribing therapy. In five eyes (four diabetics) the glaucoma was controlled after cyclotherapy, and in two eyes in which we assumed emulsification as the cause we planned to remove the oil shortly thereafter hoping that the pressure then settled. Fistulating procedures were not necessary in any of our patients. We observed glaucomatous cupping of the optic nerve head twice; one instance this prompted us to remove the silicone oil which resulted in redetachment – the eye was assigned to the failure group. In the other instance the glaucoma settled spontaneously after silicone oil removal. This patient (high myopia and giant tear) later developed a glaucoma in the unoperated eye which was difficult to control.

Secondary glaucoma after silicone oil surgery is a serious problem of largely unknown origin, a problem which evidently was well controllable in our patients, however, with unknown long-term problems. PDR and high myopia seem to constitute the most important risk factors.

#### 3.3.2.4 Rubeosis Iridis

Rubeosis iridis is a complication of vasoproliferative diseases and is said to occur occasionally after excessive retinectomy. It is a sign of a retinal ischemia as is frequently seen in PDR.

We observed a rubeosis iridis in 33 of the 350 successfully operated on eyes (9%), in 15 eyes existing preoperatively, and in 18 eyes developing postoperatively. Of these 33 patients, 27 were diabetics; among the other diagnoses rubeosis was rarely found.

Of the 96 successfully operated diabetics, 13 (14%) already had a rubeosis preoperatively. It receded spontaneously in five of those, persisted five times without causing significant problems, and in three eyes a neovascular glaucoma developed which had to be treated with cyclotherapy.

A rubeosis de novo developed postoperatively in 14 of the 96 successfully operated on diabetics (15%). In two, cyclotherapy was necessary; the remaining ones did not develop further complications. In eight of these 14 eyes the rubeosis even regressed spontaneously or disappeared completely.

All in all we saw a neovascular glaucoma in need of cyclotherapy in five of 96 successfully operated on diabetic eyes (5%). These five eyes had normal intraocular pressures at the last follow-up examination.

The incidence of rubeosis was somewhat higher among the diabetic failures: 23% had a rubeosis preoperatively and another 13% developed a new one postoperatively. Neovascular glaucoma occurred in 18% of the eyes.

There were two eyes with PVR that had rubeosis preoperatively. In one patient it disappeared after retinal reattachment, in the other patient the follow-up time was too short to assess the development. Two other patients developed rubeosis iridis postoperatively, in one patient after a peripheral retinectomy of 300°. In both patients the rubeosis regressed. A neovascular glaucoma did not develop in any of the eyes with PVR.

Rubeosis with attached retina also occurred in an eye with a giant tear and in an eye with Eales' disease. In the latter, an uncontrollable neovascular glaucoma developed.

Among the diabetic eyes the rate of newly developed rubeosis and neovascular glaucoma was surprisingly low in spite of an unfavorable preoperative situation of 14% of eyes already having preexisting rubeosis. It can be deduced from these figures that silicone oil probably inhibits the development of rubeosis and particularly of neovascular glaucoma. In other indication groups rubeosis rarely occurred and was of little clinical significance except for the eye with Eales' disease. A frequent occurrence of rubeosis after extensive retinectomy could not be found.

### 3.3.2.5 Keratopathy

Keratopathies after silicone oil surgery are divided into two forms: band keratopathy, with otherwise clear cornea and diffuse bullous keratopathy (see Color Plate 4, Figs. 2a + b). The two forms can appear in combination and probably develop by different mechanisms. In the general analysis we considered them together; a detailed breakdown can be found in Fig. 25.

The rate of keratopathy by life table analysis was 7% after 6 months and 10% after 2 years among the 350 successfully operated on eyes. As keratopathies preexisted in 2% of patients, this means that 8% developed anew. The life table curves for keratopathy in the successfully operated on eyes are shown in Fig. 24.

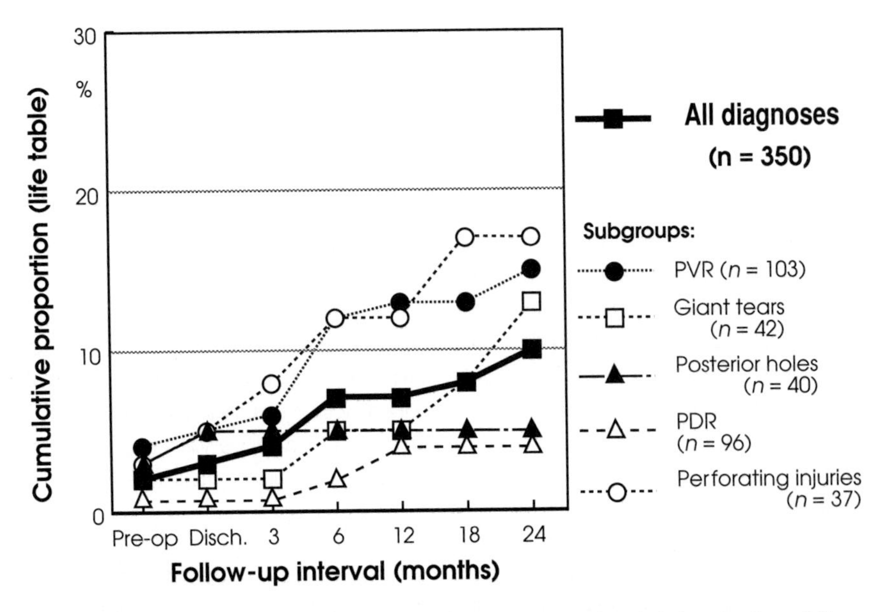


**Fig. 24.** Keratopathy in eyes with attached retina for the total cohort and those eyes with the most important well-defined clinical pictures (life table analysis)

Patients with perforating injuries showed the highest incidence of keratopathy. This was explained by the frequent involvement of the anterior segment in the trauma and the high incidence of hypotony with silicone oil prolapse into the anterior chamber in severely injured eyes. Keratopathy occurred most rarely in diabetics since we usually retained the lens for a long time, which is good protection for the anterior segment.

The keratopathy rate among the anatomic failures was much higher and amounted to 24% after 2 years (life table). This can be explained by the fact that band keratopathies occur more frequently anyway – even without silicone oil – in eyes with persisting retinal detachment. In addition hypotony as well as retinal detachment may cause silicone oil to prolapse into the anterior chamber with consequent damage to the cornea.

It is widely accepted that contact between silicone oil and cornea will cause keratopathy in the long run. Accordingly, we strive to keep the anterior chamber free of silicone oil. For this purpose we started using inferior basal iridectomies in all aphakic eyes in the beginning of 1984, the hope being that the incidence of keratopathy could be lowered significantly by this measure. In order to examine the validity of this action and to find out in what particular circumstances silicone oil prolapse caused keratopathy,

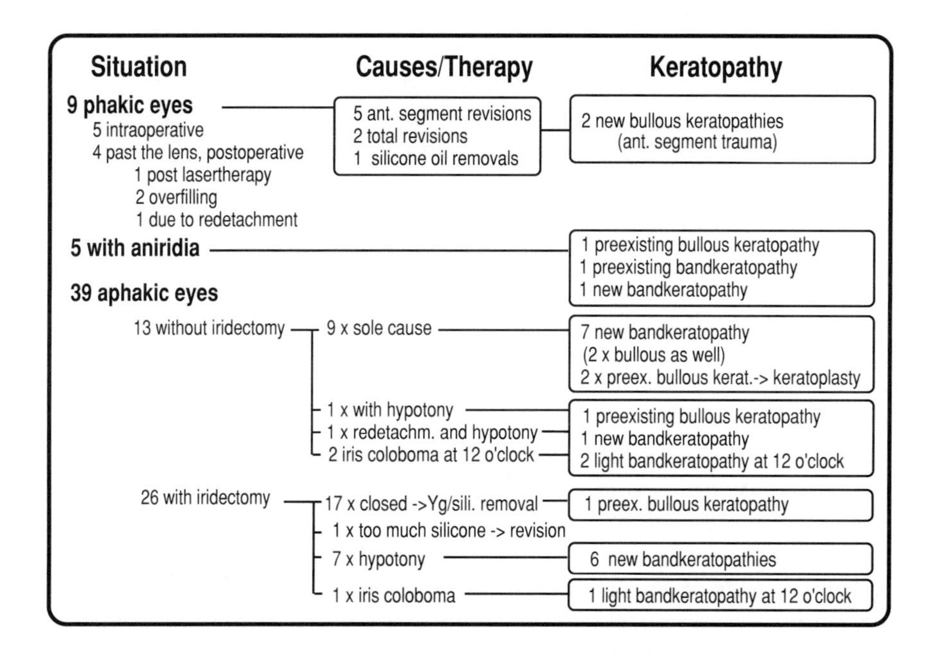


**Fig. 25.** Silicone oil prolapse into the anterior chamber and subsequent keratopathy

the fate of all eyes in which contact between silicone oil and cornea was documented is summarized in Fig. 25.

Silicone oil can contact the corneal endothelium in three basic anatomic situations: firstly in phakic eyes by prolapsing past the lens through the zonula, secondly – virtually obligatory – in eyes with aniridia or a large coloboma of the iris, and thirdly in aphakic eyes through the pupil when the iridectomy at the 6 o'clock meridian is closed or absent.

In *phakic eyes* silicone oil in the anterior chamber will not lead to keratopathy if the oil is removed again in time. Only two of the nine eyes concerned (Fig. 25) developed keratopathy, and in both instances factors other than silicone oil had at least a share in the damage to the corneal endothelium (intracapsular cataract operation in one case, and long-acting intraocular gas filling in the other one).

Keratopathy did not develop in all patients with *aniridia* either. Two of the eyes in our series had a keratopathy from the onset and two eyes did not develop a keratopathy in spite of aniridia. In the latter, the silicone oil was later removed (after 7 and 21 months, respectively).

*Aphakic eyes without iridectomy* at the 6 o'clock meridian can get spontaneous silicone oil prolapse into the anterior chamber due to the mechanism described earlier (p. 33). This happened in nine of 13 aphakic eyes. Two of them already had preexisting corneal damage, the remaining seven all developed keratopathy. These seven eyes (see Fig. 25) would probably not have developed keratopathy if we had carried out an inferior basal iridectomy at the time. In the remaining four eyes without iridectomy the endothelial contact was caused by hypotony, redetachment or iris coloboma and could probably not have been avoided by such an iridectomy.

In 26 *aphakic eyes with iridectomy* at the 6 o'clock meridian silicone oil prolapse occurred in spite of it. In 17 eyes this was caused by closure of the iridectomy due to fibrin or reproliferation, and the iridectomy had to be reopened surgically or with the Nd:Yg laser. None of these eyes developed a keratopathy. In seven eyes the silicone oil prolapse was kept up by hypotony in spite of an open iridectomy. In the further course of events six of these eyes developed a band keratopathy. Another eye, with an iris coloboma at 12 o'clock, developed a light keratopathy of the upper cornea.

A close study of Fig. 25 shows that not every silicone oil prolapse necessarily leads to keratopathy if the silicone oil is removed from the anterior chamber in time. Our data are, however, not sufficient to make statements about the length of time silicone oil is tolerated in the anterior chamber without causing damage. The clinical impression is that it is tolerated by most eyes for several weeks without permanent damage. This analysis also shows that by introducing an inferior basal iridectomy in aphakic eyes the development of keratopathy can be prevented without exception unless hypotony, redetachment, or iris coloboma coexist. These iridectomies, however, close frequently and have to be reopened, but in every instance where this happened, keratopathy could be prevented by early revision. A comparison of keratopathy rates with or without inferior basal iridectomy is shown in Fig. 27.

On the whole the incidence of keratopathy could be considerably reduced by an improved understanding of the mechanism of development and by prevention of keratopathy. Whereas in the early group 11% of the successfully operated on eyes developed a new keratopathy by 2 years, this rate was reduced to 5% in the late group.

#### 3.3.2.6 Other Complications

*Endophthalmitis* occurred in one eye after silicone oil injection. The eye had a double perforating foreign body injury with a tooth from a circular saw intraretinally. This could only be removed 9 days after the event. As the retina was severely injured, the eye was filled with silicone oil. Postoperatively the view to the posterior segment was hindered by progressive cataract, but after a few days fibrin formation in the retinal periphery became visible. The inflammation in the anterior and the posterior segments increased continuously in spite of massive therapy. At revision surgery the sclera and the retina were found to be necrotic.The eye was later enucleated. The causative agent could not be identified.

In two eyes we saw a *scleral fistula* at the temporal upper sclerotomy causing temporary hypotony. In one eye it could be resutured successfully, in the other, caused by premature removal of sutures, several unsuccessful attempts at revision were made. Both applying dural patches and the use of fibrin adhesive proved unsuccessful; eventually the fistula closed spontaneously by granulation.

*Hypotony* was a rare complication, which we observed in 17 of the 350 successfully operated on eyes. It was the consequence of damage to the ciliary body by trauma, proliferative disease in the vitreous base, string syndrome, endophthalmitis, acute retinal necrosis, or Eales' disease. In four eyes it occurred after silicone oil removal; in two eyes we therefore reinjected the silicone oil. As it was a disease-related complication, we have not analyzed hypotony in detail.

## 3.4 Influence of Special Factors on Results and Complications

### 3.4.1 Aphakia

A comparison of success and complication rates in phakic and aphakic eyes is important in the discussion of whether an early lens extraction is advisable or not. Two groups of eyes were compared: 239 eyes of our series were phakic as long as the oil was in the eye; the lens so far has not been removed, or alternatively it was extracted simultaneously with or after silicone oil removal. 235 eyes were aphakic at some time while the oil was in the eye. For this comparison we excluded 9 eyes with aniridia as they constitute a special problem. Success- and complication rates in the two groups are shown in Fig. 26a, b.

The success rates in the two samples were virtually identical at 70% (life table) after 2 years (Fig. 26a). The visual success rates and the proportions of eyes having preserved ambulatory vision (not graphically represented) also differed by less than 3 percentage points at all follow-up intervals.

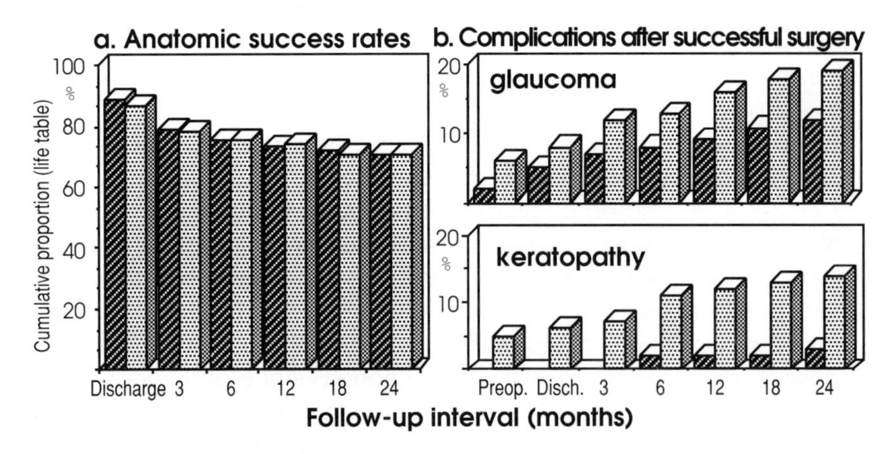


**Fig. 26a, b.** Success (**a**) and complication (**b**) rates in phakic and aphakic eyes. ▨ phakic eyes, $n = 239$; ▤ aphakic eyes, $n = 235$

The difference in complication rates, however, is substantial, at least with respect to keratopathy. In Fig. 26b, only eyes with anatomic success were evaluated. Those were 173 phakic and 170 aphakic eyes (aniridia was excluded). By life table analysis the incidence of glaucoma was 12% after 2 years in the phakic group. With 2% having a preexisting glaucoma the rate of newly developed glaucoma amounted to 10%. In the group of aphakic eyes the incidence of glaucoma was 19% after 2 years, with a growth rate of 13%.

None of the eyes in the phakic group had a preoperative keratopathy; at the end of 24 months 3% had developed one. In the aphakic group the preoperative rate was 5% and the growth rate 9%.

We did not find aphakia to have a positive influence on anatomic success even though a thorough dissection of the vitreous base can only be performed in aphakic eyes. With regard to the complication rates, however, it seems to be of definite advantage to preserve the lens as long as possible.

## 3.4.2 Inferior Basal Iridectomy ("Ando Iridectomy")

As pointed out earlier (p. 33), we started to perform an inferior basal iridectomy in aphakic eyes at the beginning of 1984, and it was apparent that contact between silicone oil and cornea could thus be avoided. One should expect therefore that with such iridectomies fewer keratopathies,

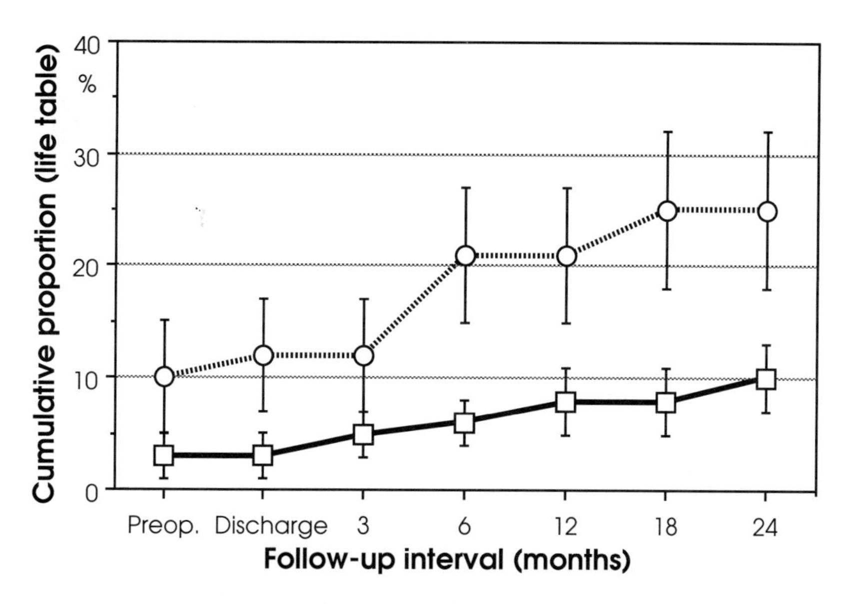


**Fig. 27.** Influence of the inferior basal iridectomy on the incidence of keratopathy in aphakic eyes with attached retina. ⋯○⋯ without inferior basal iridectomy ($n$ = 50); —□— with inferior basal iridectomy ($n$ = 120); *Error bars* 1 standard deviation

fewer early pupil- or angle-block situations, and, as a consequence, perhaps fewer cases of late glaucoma will develop.

Altogether 120 of the eyes successfully operated on received such an iridectomy. Another 50 aphakic eyes with attached retinas were operated on before introduction of iridectomy.

The rates of keratopathy in these two samples are shown in Fig. 27.

The incidence of keratopathy without iridectomy was 25% in aphakic eyes at 2 years; the growth rate was about 15%. With iridectomy the incidence declined to 10% and the growth rate (7%) was practically halved. These figures reflect that keratopathies in aphakic eyes are avoidable if the iris diaphragm is intact and no hypotony is present.

It appears that early pupil- or angle-block situations with raised intraocular pressures were controlled better since the introduction of the inferior iridectomy. As the iridectomies, however, often occluded spontaneously, such situations have probably not become very much rarer. The data are, however, not sufficient to support this impression statistically.

An analysis of the rates of *persisting glaucoma* showed that the incidence of glaucoma increased considerably after the introduction of the inferior basal iridectomy (Fig. 28).

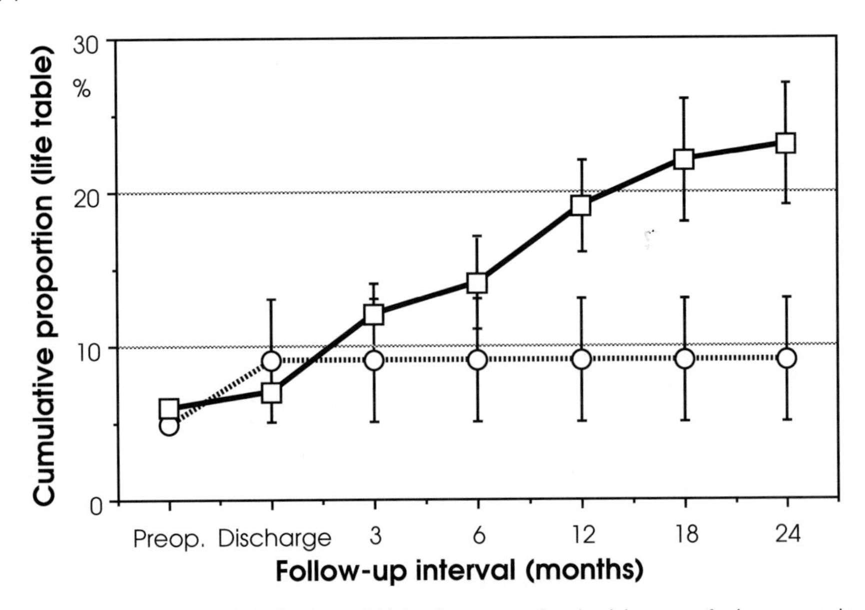


**Fig. 28.** Influence of inferior basal iridectomy on the incidence of glaucoma in aphakic eyes with attached retinas. ⋯○⋯ without inferior basal iridectomy ($n$ = 50); —□— with inferior basal iridectomy ($n$ = 120); *Error bars* 1 standard deviation

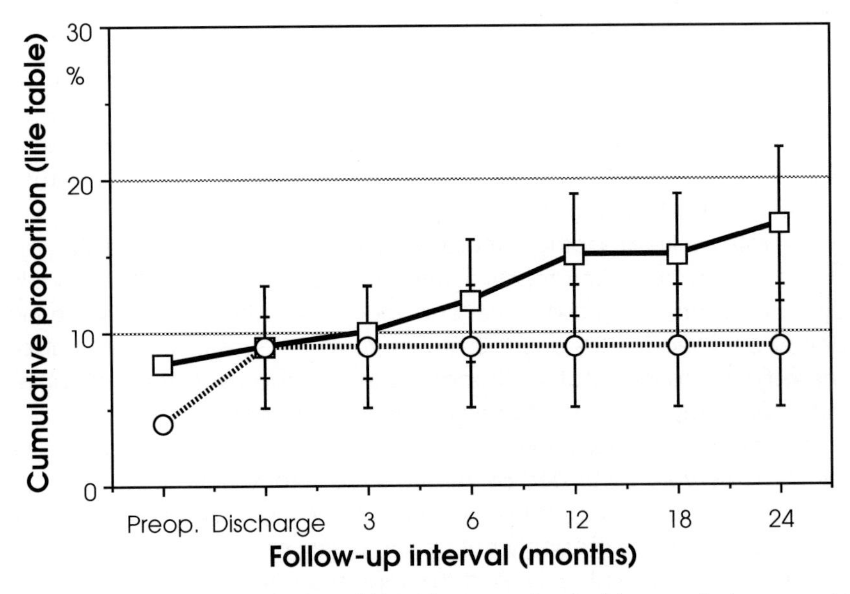


**Fig. 29.** Influence of inferior basal iridectomy on the incidence of glaucoma in aphakic eyes with attached retina (all indication groups except diabetes). ⋯○⋯ without inferior basal iridectomy ($n$ = 50); —□— with inferior basal iridectomy ($n$ = 120); *Error bars* 1 standard deviation

This was surprising at first and did not correspond to the clinical expectation that chronic late glaucoma may sometimes be avoided by eliminating early angle-block situations. An explanation for this high glaucoma rate is found in the fact that there was a considerably higher proportion of diabetics with neovascular glaucoma among the eyes operated on with a 6 o'clock iridectomy. If we disregard diabetics in the analysis of glaucoma rates and only consider the remaining indication groups, the difference between the glaucoma rates with and without 6 o'clock iridectomy is no longer so high (Fig. 29).

There still remained a somewhat higher incidence of glaucoma in the eyes *with* inferior iridectomy for which we could not find an explanation. It must be taken into consideration, however, that due to the relatively small sample size the differences in Fig. 29 are statistically not highly significant. A positive influence of the inferior basal iridectomy on glaucoma could not be demonstrated, however.

### 3.4.3 Silicone Oil Removal

We have meanwhile removed the silicone oil in 168 of the 350 successfully operated on eyes. To determine the influence of silicone oil removal on the incidence of complications, we compared this sample of eyes, in which the proportion with intraocular silicone oil became smaller from interval to interval and in which the oil is finally removed from all eyes at the end of the follow-up period, with a control group, in which, at the time of the last examination, the oil was still in the eye. The average length of follow-up was, of course, longer in the group with oil removal (28 months) than in the control group (17 months) (Fig. 30).

In the group in which the silicone oil was removed, the incidence of glaucoma (26%) after 2 years was considerably higher than in the control group (10%). In both groups 4% of the eyes had preoperative glaucoma. The relative increase in keratopathies was roughly the same in both groups, 6% and 8%, respectively.

These figures could lead one to conclude that the incidence of glaucoma was lowered by removing the silicone oil, whereas the incidence of keratopathy remained unaffected. This conclusion is, however, invalid since the groups analyzed are statistically not comparable. Such a comparison would only be valid if the decision for silicone oil removal had been randomized and not made on the basis of clinical criteria. It is fair to assume that many of the eyes in which the silicone oil was left beyond 24 months had more complicated problems on the whole, which by themselves might have been responsible for a higher rate of glaucoma.

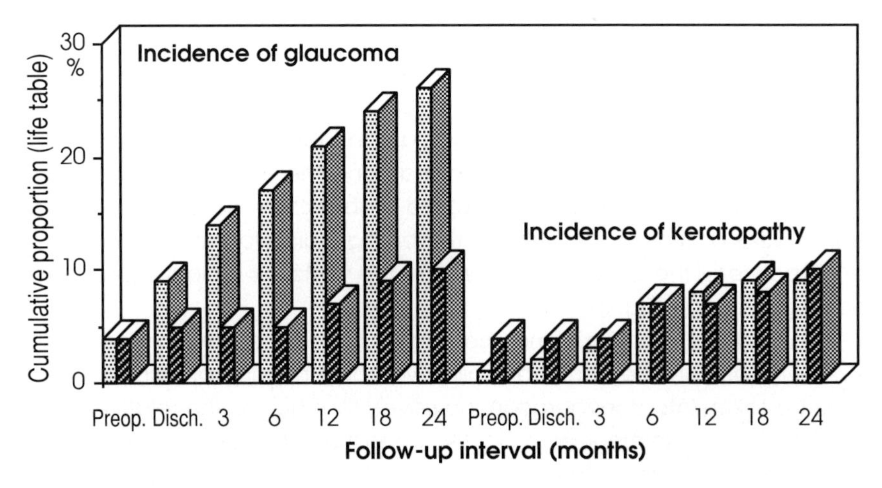


**Fig. 30.** Influence of silicone oil removal on the incidence of glaucoma and keratopathy in eyes with attached retinas. ▒ without silicone removal ($n$ = 182); ▨ with silicone removal ($n$ = 168)

## 3.4.4 Retinectomy

Retinotomies and retinectomies are used to drain subretinal fluid, remove subretinal strands, and relieve retinal traction. We frequently performed smaller drainage retinotomies without observing serious complications in the process. They will therefore not be analyzed any further.

We have compared eyes with and without retinectomy in the two indication groups in which retinectomies were performed to any extent (PVR and PDR) in order to examine whether there was any influence of larger retinal cuts on the success rates.

We operated on 50 eyes with PVR, performing a large retinectomy, whereas in another 94 cases this maneuver did not seem necessary. With PDR the corresponding figures were 34 eyes with and 102 eyes without retinectomy. The anatomic success rates by life table analysis are shown in Fig. 31.

The success rates in PVR were virtually the same for both the subgroup without retinectomy (69% after 2 years) and the one with retinectomy (64%).

In PDR the results in the group with retinectomy (62% after 2 years) were somewhat worse than in the control group (70%), but this difference was clinically not relevant.

Considering that the anatomically and pathologically more complicated eyes were probably more likely to be treated with retinectomies, these figures suggest that retinectomies had no practical negative influence on the success rates.

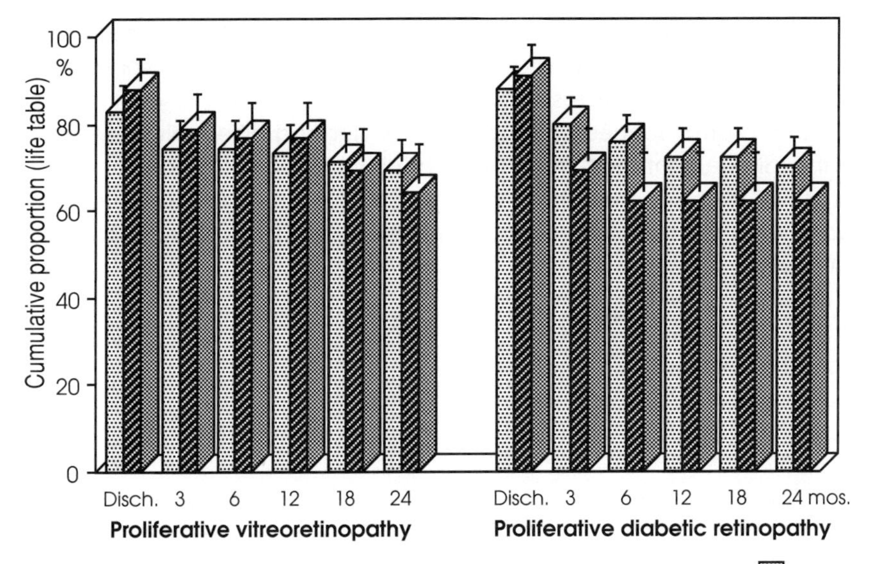


**Fig. 31.** Success rates in PVR and PDR with and without retinectomy. without retinectomy ; with retinectomy; *Error bars,* 1 standard deviation

### 3.4.5 Comparison of Surgeons

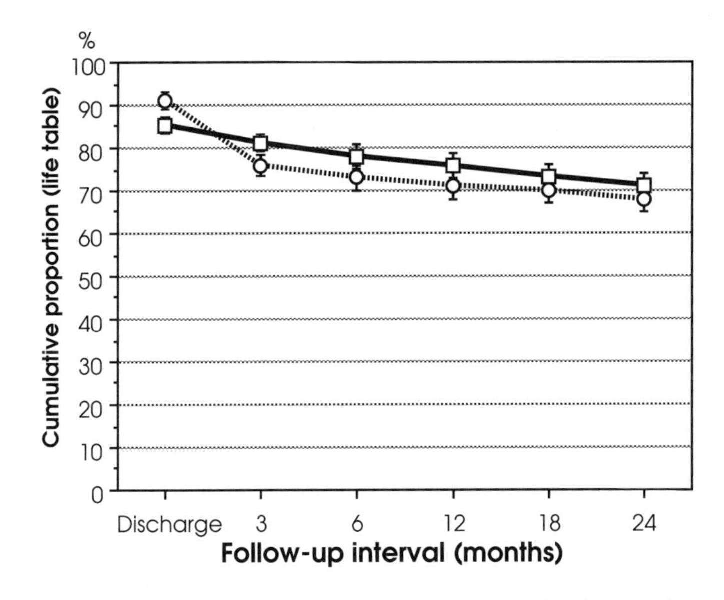


**Fig. 32.** Comparison of the anatomic success rates for the two main surgeons. surgeon 1 ($n = 254$); surgeon 2 ($n = 213$); *Error bars,* 1 standard deviation

Two surgeons operated 96.7% of the eyes analyzed in this study. Both operated on similarly large groups of eyes (254 and 213). A comparison of the anatomic success rates is shown in Fig. 32.

The anatomic success rates are very similar and differ only very slightly for the follow-up intervals from 3 months onwards. This probably shows that in spite of all the complexity extreme retinal surgery is a procedure which can lead to reproducible results if equipment and surgical techniques are the same.

# 4 Discussion

## 4.1 Results

### 4.1.1 General Aspects

#### 4.1.1.1 Problems of Analysis

The greatest problem in evaluating such a large group of eyes operated on with silicone oil was the fact that preoperative anatomic situations, surgical procedures, and postoperative clinical courses were extraordinarily variable. This is already evidenced by the fact that in the tables summarizing the results (Tables 5 and 6) the whole sample investigated had to be broken down into 24 subgroups of anywhere between 226 and 8 eyes. Complicated retinal detachments being in need of this therapy are rare, but this fact and the great heterogeneity of the initial findings make statistical evaluation very difficult. Multifactorial analyses would be ideal for the analysis of many aspects, but the number of variables is in most instances too large and the number of patients in the subgroups generally too small to facilitate statistically highly significant statements. In such situations life table analysis has established itself as the common form of analysis. We have supplemented it where necessary by individual case analyses if only a few cases existed or if additional clinical information could be gained by it.

#### 4.1.1.2 Comparability of Various Studies

The object of this study is to present data based on a large sample of patients, analyze the most pertinent questions, and if possible compare the results with those of other studies. Due to innumerable variations the latter is, however, only possible to a limited extent as the preoperative situations and the conceptional ideas of the surgeons regarding indication, surgical technique, and follow-up care differ from study to study.

The *preoperative anatomic situations*, for instance, of the patients included in such studies will probably be quite different. Depending on training and experience, temperament and courage, every surgeon will have different criteria on the basis of which a retinal detachment is classified as inoperable or in the light of which different procedures – conventional retinal surgery, vitrectomy, with gas or with silicone oil are chosen. The samples will also differ as to kind and number of previous operations performed, whether they are phakic, aphakic, or pseudophakic, have episcleral implants, encircling bands, etc. Finally, there will be preoperative factors influencing success or failure which cannot be measured.

We have tried therefore to generate subclassifications for individual clinical diagnoses to ensure better comparability of the results. The classification of PVR, as suggested by the Retina Society (1983), is a method allowing us to classify our patients with PVR based on anatomic criteria only. Unfortunately though it neglects the extremely important factor of proliferation dynamics since it cannot be measured. More recently, a similar classification has also become available for PDR (Kroll et al. 1987), but it has yet to establish itself in the literature and, analogous to the classification of PVR, it does not take the fulminance of neovascular activity into account nor does it consider the degree of preceding laser therapy and the risk factors for developing neovascular glaucoma. For the other clinical diagnoses presented here, so far no classification methods exist.

*Surgical technique* will probably also differ considerably among study groups. In such complicated procedures, lasting up to 6 h at times and comprising many single surgical steps, the surgeon must make a series of individual decisions concerning the kind of procedure and perform maneuvers which will differ depending on experience, conceptual understanding, and manual technique. Vitrectomy of the vitreous base, for instance, is performed with different degrees of care, and, for conceptional and technical reasons, there are differences as to how often and how correctly additional measures, such as encircling buckle, cryocoagulations, endolaser, and retinotomies, are carried out. The surgical equipment available also differs from one operating theater to another.

*Follow-up care* will also influence the success rates significantly. Many of these complicated cases develop renewed retinal detachment through reproliferation. Evaluation of this reproliferation and the decision on the necessity of a revision procedure aiming at stabilization will have a large bearing on eventual success. Patient guidance is of great importance. Depending on age, general health, or whether it is the only eye, it will be possible or necessary to motivate the patient in favor of or against revision surgery. The decision if and when the silicone oil must be removed also depends on many individual factors, and might therefore well be handled differently in different studies, thereby influencing the results.

Finally the *statistical methods* vary in different studies. Whereas today life table analysis has established itself for studies of samples with varying lengths of follow-up, it was common in former times to report only success rates after 6 months and to exclude patients with a shorter observation time. As we showed earlier (p. 39), this procedure would have resulted in a falsification of our results for the better. Furthermore, our results show that in the clinical conditions discussed here, with a strong tendency to reproliferation, a stable state had not been reached by 6 months at all; our anatomic success rates declined further between 6 and 24 months due to continuing proliferation. Lastly, the definition of anatomic success is not uniform in all studies. The definition of complete retinal attachment posterior to the encircling buckle, used by us and set down by the international conference of the Retina Foundation in 1962, is applied in most studies; however, in a paper published recently on success rates after surgery on eyes with complicated PVR by means of vitrectomy, perfluoropropane, and panretinal laser coagulation, reattachment of the macula was taken as the success criterion (Fisher et al. 1988).

Being aware of all these problems of comparability among various studies, in the discussion following we shall try to evaluate our results in the light of the pertinent literature.

## 4.1.2 Results by Indication Groups

### 4.1.2.1 Proliferative Vitreoretinopathy

PVR is still the most serious complication of retinal detachment and occurs in about 5% – 10% of eyes (Rachal and Burton 1979, Haimann et al. 1982, Ryan 1985a). Pigment epithelial cells, when liberated, undergo metaplasia and develop into fibroblast-like cells (Machemer and Laqua 1975). They multiply and form clumps on and under the retina, on vitreous membranes, ciliary body, iris, and the back surface of the lens. Retinal glial cells participate in the process, passing through the internal and external limiting membranes and forming sheets of cells on the retinal surfaces (Laqua and Machemer 1975). Some of these metaplastic cells contain intracytoplasmic contractile filaments which contract to cause retinal detachment. After contraction of these membranes the process is stabilized by deposition of newly formed collagen (Laqua 1981).

The final result, fixed retinal folds and tractional strands in the vitreous cavity, was called massive vitreous retraction (MVR) (Cibis 1965a), massive preretinal retraction (MPR) (Tolentino et al. 1967), or massive periretinal proliferation (MPP) (Machemer 1977) until the terminology committee of the Retina Society decided on "proliferative vitreoretinopathy" (1983) as the standard expression.

In spite of intensive research in this field for more than 20 years and the development of numerous animal models (e.g., Cleary and Ryan 1979, Topping et al. 1979, Miller et al. 1985, Zhu et al. 1988), predominantly using rabbits, there is still uncertainty as to the initiating factors and many of the pathogenetic mechanisms. A convincing pharmacological approach has not been found so far.

Before the introduction of vitreous surgery there was no promising therapy for advanced PVR. Success rates with buckling measures only amounted to about 25% – 35% for stages C2-D1; stages D2 and D3 could not be successfully treated at all (Grizzard and Hilton 1982). The first results after the introduction of pars plana vitrectomy – 36% (Machemer 1977) and 42% (Ratner et al. 1983) – were disappointing.

**Table 10**. Surgery for PVR: success rates with vitrectomy and gas

| Study (year) | PVR stage | *n* | Method | Success (%) | Follow-up (months) |
|---|---|---|---|---|---|
| Machemer, Laqua (1978c) | na | 47 | VY and air/SF6 | 36 | ≥6 |
| Laqua (unpublished) (1982) | na | 21 | VY and air/SF6 | 45 | ≥6 |
| Chang et al. (1984) | C3-D2 | 18 | VY and CnFn, Gas | 56 | ≥6 |
| Jalkh et al. (1984) | C1-D3 | 410 | VY and air | 59 | ≥6 |
| Chang et al. (1985) | C3-D3 | 20 | VY and CnFn,Gas | 60 | ≥6 |
| Ho et al. (1985) | C3-D3 | 75 | VY and air | 56 | ≥6 |
| Sternberg et al. (1985) | C1-D3 | 72 | VY and air/SF6 | 33 | ≥6 |
| Fisher et al. (1988) | C3-D3 | 76 | VY and CnFn and Laser | 65[1] | ≥12 |
| Lewis et al. (1988a) | C3-D3 | 74 | VY and CnFn | 80 | ≥6 |

VY, vitrectomy; na, not available; SF6, sulfur hexafluoride; CnFn, perfluorocarbon gas
[1]82% with attached macula

Then, in the 1980s, surgery with vitrectomy and gas was further pursued and improved upon in the USA. The results with this technique for the studies published so far are summarized in Table 10. It is surprising how much the success rates continue to vary, ranging from 33% (Sternberg and Machemer 1985) to 80% (Lewis and Aaberg 1988), even though the number of patients is approximately equal and the surgical technique allegedly basically the same as well. By including stages C1 and C2, Sternberg even included patients with a better prognosis. These differences, we think, reflect the fact that indication, surgical technique, and statistical method tend to differ widely.

Further information about possible success rates with vitrectomy and gas can be obtained from the breakdown by stages of PVR (Table 11). The success rates for the advanced stages D1-D3 can be seen to be considerably worse in almost all studies, but in spite of classification the results still vary widely.

**Table 11**. Success rates in PVR by stages: vitrectomy and gas

| | | (% Success) | | | | | |
|---|---|---|---|---|---|---|---|
| Study (year) | *n* | C1 | C2 | C3 | D1 | D2 | D3 |
| Chang et. al. (1984) | 18 | | | 100 | 75 | 25 | |
| Jalkh et. al. (1984) | 410 | 55 | 75 | 65 | 60 | 57 | 35 |
| Ho et. al. (1985) | 75 | 100 | 100 | 73 | 54 | 50 | 26 |
| Sternberg et. al. (1985) | 72 | 69 | 69 | 15 | 33 | 25 | 15 |
| Fisher et. al. (1988) | 76 | | | 86 | 68 | 60 | 27 |

Tables 12 and 13 show analogous data for all studies with silicone oil published so far and for our results. In contrast to the publications on vitrectomy and gas we find mostly European studies; only in the last few years have some American studies also been published (McCuen et al. 1985, Cox et al. 1986, Sell et al. 1897, Yeo et al. 1987, Lewis et al. 1988b).

With silicone oil a general trend to better results over the years is apparent and here too there are large differences in success rates among various authors. On the whole our results, however, are similar to those of other European silicone oil surgeons, whereas the results of some American studies possibly reflect the fact that some surgeons are still in the learning phase and are relatively inexperienced in these techniques. Summing up all published cases, there is a success rate of 54.8% for gas and 59.3% for silicone oil.

**Table 12**. Surgery for PVR: success rates with vitrectomy and silicone oil

| Study (year) | PVR stage | *n* | Method | Success (%) | Follow-up (months) |
|---|---|---|---|---|---|
| Grey et al. (1979) | na | 91 | silicone, *no* VY | 55 | 12 |
| Živojnović et al. (1982) | all | 280 | VY and silicone | 57 | ≥2 years |
| Laqua et al. (1982) | na | 61 | VY and silicone | 63 | 12 |
| Gonvers (1982a) | C3-D3 | 21 | VY and temp. silic. | 57 | 6 |
| Diddie et al. (1983) | C1-D3 | 20 | VY and silicone | 30 | ≥6 |
| Gnad et al. (1984) | na | 28 | VY and silicone | 42 | ≥6 |
| Heimann et al. (1984b) | na | 143 | VY and silicone | 53 | 6 |
| Gonvers (1985) | C1-D3 | 146 | VY and temp. silic. | 62 | 6 |
| McCuen et al. (1985) | C2-D3 | 44 | VY and silicone | 64 | ≥6 |
| Tavakolian et al. (1985) | na | 100 | VY and silicone | 52 | ≥6 |
| Cox et al. (1986) | D1-D3 | 51 | VY and silicone | 51 | ≥6 |
| Sell et al. (1987) | C2-D3 | 47 | VY and silicone | 74 | 6 |
| Yeo et al. (1987) | C3-D3 | 30 | VY and silicone | 67 | ≥6 |
| Lewis and Aaberg (1988b) | C3-D3 | 31 | VY and silicone | 67 | ≥6 |
| Binder et al. (1988a) | C3-D3 | 44 | VY and silicone | 61 | ≥10 |
| *This study (1990)* | PVR C1-D3 | 144 | VY and Silicone | 75 | 6[1] |

VY, vitrectomy; na, not available
[1]life table analysis

**Table 13**. Success rates in PVR by stages: vitrectomy and silicone oil

| Study (year) | n | (% Success) C1 | C2 | C3 | D1 | D2 | D3 |
|---|---|---|---|---|---|---|---|
| Gonvers (1985) | 146 | 80 | 81 | 64 | 54 | 47 | 45 |
| McCuen et al. (1985) | 44 | | 75 | 67 | 36 | 19 | 43 |
| Cox et al. (1986) | 51 | | | | 67 | 69 | 50 |
| *This study (1990)* | 144 | 88 | 81 | 65 | 89 | 66 | 75 |

The differences between gas and silicone oil become more distinct if analyzed by PVR stages. Unfortunately, there are only a few publications on gas or on silicone in which these stages are broken down. Thus only relatively small numbers of cases are available for analysis. It is also remarkable that our results for the advanced stages D1-D3 are considerably better than those of other surgeons using silicone oil (Gonvers 1985, McCuen et al. 1985, Cox et al. 1985). To understand this, it is important to know that Gonvers removed the silicone oil in all his patients after 4–6 weeks and did not perform revision surgery on redetachments. Both McCuen and Cox operated only on those eyes with silicone oil that had been operated on without success with gas before. This could very well have resulted in a negative selection. In spite of all this, if the results for gas and silicone oil are compared (Tables 11 and 13), we get published average success rates of 75% with gas and 80% with silicone oil for stage C, but 42% with gas and 60% with silicone oil for stage D. Although these studies are hardly comparable, a trend is noticeable here which coincides with clinical experience: For the advanced stages of PVR the success rates with silicone oil are probably considerably better than those with gas, an opinion which by now is shared by most American surgeons (see Color Plate 1, Figs 1a + b).

The main cause for failure is *reproliferation* of pre- and occasionally also subretinal membranes. A comparison of our results for PVR between the early and the late group showed that the rates of redetachment between discharge from hospital and 24 months later remained unchanged over the course of the years. In almost all our patients this could be attributed to reproliferation. The rate of loss amounted to 16% in both the early group and in the late one. The better anatomic long-term results achieved in the late group were due to better attachment rates at the time of discharge (92% as compared to 73%), i.e., probably a result of improved surgical technique.

In the beginning there was widespread hope that silicone oil might be able to prevent reproliferation. Meanwhile several animal experimental studies have reached contradictory results on this question.

In a fibroblast model using rabbits Gonvers (1983) found that in eyes filled with silicone oil the detachment rate was reduced by 50% as compared to the control group. Above all there was less contraction of epiretinal star folds. After perforating injury Lemmen et al. (1988b) found a 100% rate of traction detachment in rabbit eyes filled with gas and saline, whereas the majority of the eyes filled with silicone oil did not develop retinal detachment.

Leon et al. (1984) and Fastenberg et al. (1983), however, came to opposite results. In their fibroblast models with silicone oil they found proliferation patterns and detachment rates not different from those of the control groups without silicone oil.

After injecting pigment epithelial cells Lambrou et al. (1987) found the highest detachment rates in eyes filled with silicone oil. Moreover in aspirates taken from the remaining vitreous they showed that fluid taken from eyes with silicone oil had higher mitogenic activity in culture on pigmentepithelial cells than on controls. They came to the conclusion that the silicone oil must be responsible for this high mitogenic activity. They speculated that, on the one hand, the concentration of proliferative factors in the narrow space between silicone oil bubble and retina might have been responsible for this increase in activity. On the other hand, however, silicone oil itself may have stimulated the release of growth factors or acted directly as a mitogen.

The reasons for these contradictory experimental results demonstrating positive as well as negative influences of silicone oil on proliferative activity remain unclear. The experiments by Lambrou et al. have doubtlessly directed the attention to clinically visible reproliferations ("perisilicone proliferation", Lewis et al. 1988). These were already known and were considered to be a continuation of the proliferative process active preoperatively; however, they are now suspected of being caused by the silicone oil directly.

It is difficult to answer the question clinically whether silicone oil stimulates such proliferation or simply does not prevent it, as the patterns of reproliferation are known but cannot be measured quantitatively. Accordingly, disagreement exists on how to interpret these reproliferations. The consequence is that different authors can arrive at diametrically opposed conclusions as to the significance of reproliferation by using different evaluation criteria (Foerster et al. 1988 and Kroll et al. 1988b).

Our redetachment rate through reproliferation (66% in the late group) was actually even higher than that of Lewis et al. (1988), who observed such reproliferations in 61% of their 31 patients with PVR. The proliferations eventually caused redetachment in 49% of all their patients operated on with silicone oil. Corresponding figures on reproliferation and redetachment have unfortunately never been published by American surgeons operating with gas. As the success rates with gas are generally lower than those with silicone oil, at least for the advanced stages of PVR, it must be assumed that these can hardly be lower. Besides, certain proliferation patterns, e.g., fibrotic membranes in the vitreous base, which once were regarded as characteristic of eyes filled with silicone oil, have meanwhile also been described in eyes that were treated with long-acting gas tamponade (Hutten 1988). It seems therefore that these new proliferation patterns are more typical of long-term tamponade in general and less an effect caused by silicone oil specifically.

It is our clinical impression, based on the eyes we operated on with gas, that the redetachment rates with gas are probably higher than with silicone oil. Above all, eyes operated on with gas after resorption of the bubble can end up much more quickly in an inoperable condition than eyes with silicone oil. Growth behavior of newly developing membranes is clinically different in eyes filled with silicone oil from that after gas surgery and corresponds to the model found by Gonvers in his rabbit experiment (1983a). The membranes grow flatter, their ability to form star folds is probably reduced due to a mechanical effect of the silicone oil bubble, and they are less able to contract the retina. By tamponading the rhegmatogenous component, renewed retinal detachments remain more limited in their extent and an additional stimulation of the proliferative process is thus eliminated. Repeat surgery becomes easier, and it can be delayed until the proliferative process has slowed down. In such a situation, with only little or no proliferative activity still present, chances of reattaching the retina permanently by a revision operation are considerably improved. This is corroborated by the fact that we were able to reattach the retina permanently in 78% of all eyes redetaching after a primarily successful silicone oil operation (p. 43). Only 10% of the eyes primarily successfully operated on actually reached an inoperable condition due to reproliferation.

A further clinical argument against the hypothesis that silicone oil might stimulate proliferation is the low rate of proliferation found in eyes with uncomplicated giant tears and posterior holes. The natural untreated course in these eyes, particularly with giant tears, leads almost inevitably to massive PVR. After silicone oil injection we saw membrane formation in only 24% of the eyes overall; in only 10% did the redetachment develop because of membrane formation. If the natural course in eyes with giant tears leads to PVR and the hypothesis that silicone oil stimulates proliferation is correct, it is hard to understand why our rate of redetachment due to proliferative membrane formation in giant tears was so low.

Histologically, there was also no evidence supporting the stimulation hypothesis. Membranes which we removed from eyes filled with silicone oil differed from membranes taken from eyes without silicone oil only by the additional feature of vacuoles, which probably contained silicone oil droplets (see Color Plate 3, Fig 2b). Differences regarding cell or growth characteristics were not found (Bornfeld et al. 1987). Ultimately only direct comparison between gas and silicone oil in randomized, comparable patient groups can attempt to answer the questions of reproliferation and complication rates in silicone oil and gas surgery. Such a study will incur considerable expense and, due to the inhomogeneity of the initial pathologies, it will be extremely difficult to compile sufficiently large patient samples for statistically significant results.

With regard to our relatively good success rates with silicone oil, considerable ethical objections to such a study could be put forward. Such a multicentric study is, however, presently being carried out in the USA (Ryan 1985b). The result is eagerly awaited.

The question as to whether silicone oil inhibits or stimulates proliferation cannot yet be answered clearly. Animal experiments are as contradictory as the clinical studies published. In eyes filled with silicone oil we doubtlessly saw proliferation patterns that were previously unknown (see Color Plate 3, Fig 2a). On the retina they often already appeared within a few weeks and constituted a complication that could be controlled by revision surgery. In the vitreous base they were usually only found after many months and it was unclear whether this would cause more serious problems in the long run. For this reason and for others we decided to remove silicone oil whenever it seemed feasible. As a rule we performed this after about 12 months (Fig. 20).

The problem of reproliferation, discussed here in the context of PVR, can similarly be found in other indication groups.

#### 4.1.2.2 Giant tears

For a long time giant tears have confronted retinal surgeons with great problems. A giant tear is defined as a mostly equatorial retinal tear with an extension of at least 90°. The vitreous body is usually firmly attached to the anterior remnant of retina, and it has produced the giant tear by traction. The posterior part of the retina is folded over so that usually the underside of the retina can be visualized at ophthalmoscopy. The central folded over retina is caught in the vitreous scaffold.

The surgical problems comprise firstly mobilization of the retina, secondly unfolding, and thirdly fixation in the anatomically correct position. Before the days of vitrectomy, most surgical attempts failed because it was virtually impossible to fold back the retina and bring the retinal edge onto the buckle, particularly with more extensive tears (Table 14). Schepens and Freeman (1967) achieved a success rate of 61% in their series of giant tears, but this was reduced to only 14% for tears larger than 180°. Norton et al. (1969) (63% total success, 0% if more than 180°), Wessing et al. (1974) (50% total success, 11% if more than 180°), and Kanski (1975) (58% total success, 11% if more than 180°) fared similarly.

With the introduction of vitrectomy the problem of *mobilization* was solved. Machemer et al. (1969 and 1976) showed that even giant tears of more than 180° could be attached with vitrectomy and gas; their primary success rates (1976) amounted to 86%. The procedure involved extraordinary measures, however, such as rotating operating tables. In addition the surgeon had to kneel on the floor underneath the patient during gas injection so that the gas bubble could unfold the retina from below. Enthusiasm because of the surgical success was dampened, however, by a 42% redetachment rate resulting from secondary PVR (also see: Freeman and Castillejos 1981: 58% PVR; Laqua and Wessing 1983: 65%; Ratner et al. 1983: 35%). Nonetheless Machemer wrote at the time that the surgical problems had been solved, the remaining objective was to prevent membrane formation.

Other surgeons, however, had still other problems with this method. The main difficulty was the inability to drain the subretinal liquid completely and to press the retina onto the pigment epithelium exactly where it belonged. It often slipped to the posterior pole due to gas pressure, clumped there, and the retinal edge could not be cryopexied at the anatomically correct site. Thus, to *fixate the retinal edge*, methods were devised which had already been partly developed in earlier days and seemed suitable, particularly in gas surgery, to fixate all kinds of larger retinal defects such as giant tears and retinectomies.

Howard and Gaasterland (1970), Fung et al. (1974), Michels et al. (1983), and Peyman et al. (1984) recommended, for instance, to *incarcerate* retina or vitreous body in the sclera. This method was temporarily applied with or without silicone oil in Europe (Heimann 1980, Laqua and Wessing 1983). We performed incarcerations in 15 eyes with giant tears from 1981 to the end of 1983. It was technically very difficult and time consuming, there was always the danger of provoking massive hemorrhages, and it was not always easy to pull the correct part of the retinal edge to the sclerotomy site. In spite of this 12 of the 15 giant tears could be successfully attached by this method. Nine of these 15 giant tears were 180° or larger, including four that exceeded 270°.

Others tried to *sew the retina on* (Usui et al. 1979, Federmann et al. 1982), an idea that goes back to Galezowski (1890) and was also applied by Scott (1974) and Živojnović (personal communication) within the context of silicone oil surgery. Others developed *magnetic systems* (Lobel et al. 1978, Eckardt and Hennig 1984), with the help of which the retina could be held onto the pigment epithelium intraoperatively. This procedure was technically too difficult as well and too pregnant with complications to be able to establish itself in the long run.

"*Retinal tacking*" established itself widely as a fixation method. It is still being used in many centers especially in the USA. In this procedure described by Ando and Kondo in 1983, the retinal edge is pinned onto the choroid with small 3 mm tacks of plastic, metal, or ceramic. Others (de Juan et al. 1985+1986a, Abrams et al. 1986, Burke et al. 1987, Lewis et al. 1987b, and O'Grady et al. 1988) have refined the method and reported on their experiences with it. After giving up the incarceration method we used retinal tacks in four eyes, and soon found out that there was little use for them in silicone oil surgery. Silicone oil surgery has made all fixation aids superfluous as the silicone oil itself can be used effectively as an aid to manipulate and fixate the retina (Fig. 5). In addition it seems to reduce PVR problems postoperatively.

Laqua and Wessing published their comparative results of three surgical methods in 1983 (Table 14). They showed that, with vitrectomy and gas, 43% of the retinas could be attached initially, but that the final success rate amounted to only 28%. Using the incarceration method additionally the primary rate of attachment could be increased to 91%, but because of PVR the final success rate went down to 50%. Only by introducing silicone oil could satisfactory long-term results be achieved: The primary success rate was 87% and the final one 67%.

Table 14 shows that the best results were achieved by applying silicone oil. In our group of patients evaluated here, two eyes with giant tears were

**Table 14:** Success Rates in the Surgery of Giant Tears

| Study (year) | *n* | Method | Success rate (%) total | >180° |
|---|---|---|---|---|
| Schepens et al. (1967) | 47 | EB, gas | 61 | 14 |
| Machemer et al. (1969) | 26 | EB, gas | 65 | 25 |
| Norton et al. (1969) | 27 | EB, gas | 63 | 0 |
| Wessing et al. (1974) | 74 | excentric EB | 50 | 11 |
| Kanski (1975) | 95 | EB (19x IC) | 58 | 11 |
| Machemer et al. (1976) | 14 | EB, VY, gas | | 42 |
| Freeman et al. (1981) | 78 | EB, VY, gas | 46 | 48 |
| Lean et al. (1982) | 42 | EB, VY, Si | 88 | |
| Laqua, Wessing (1983) | 14 | EB, VY, gas | 28 | |
| Laqua, Wessing (1983) | 12 | EB, VY, IC, gas | 50 | |
| Laqua, Wessing (1983) | 24 | EB, VY, IC, Si | 67 | |
| Billington et al. (1986) | 65 | EB, VY, Si | 83 | |
| *this study (1990)* | 45 | EB, VY, Si | 93 | 100 |

EB, encircling band; VY, vitrectomy; IC, incarcerations; Si, silicone oil primary failures due to massive choroidal hemorrhage. A third, heavily traumatized eye failed as a consequence of the original surgical trauma. All other uncomplicated giant tears, i.e., without preoperative PVR, could be reattached successfully (see Color Plate 1, Figs. 2a + b).

For the sake of completeness the fate of 20 giant tears combined with PVR shall be mentioned. There were 11 that could be attached successfully. Of the other nine eyes, five were primary failures; seven (all after trauma) developed massive reproliferation. Here too in a very complicated set of patients, the rate of reproliferation was relatively low and, besides, almost exclusively associated with trauma.

In this group of eyes we were able to improve our technique over the course of time as well: Eight of the nine failures were treated in the years 1981-1983. Since May 1983, only one giant tear with PVR has been treated without success.

We had to perform revision operations 17 times in the 42 successful giant tears. Quite different from the eyes with PVR the cause was only rarely reproliferation (four times: p. 44). In ten eyes new tear formation in areas outside the original giant tear made repeat surgery necessary. Some of these new tears appeared a fairly long time after silicone oil removal. Greater attention should therefore be paid to these areas. We recommend that eyes with giant tears generally be treated with an encircling band and coagulated circumferentially, including those areas with attached retina. Nonetheless, we saw among our giant tears two eyes with massive choroidal detachment, two with string syndrome, and one with a subretinal hemorrhage after extensive cryocoagulation. The recommendation above must therefore be modified and a careful, possibly step-by-step procedure is advised in highly myopic eyes at risk of developing such complications.

In contrast to our good anatomical results there were, unfortunately, eight patients that in spite of good retinal attachment did not achieve ambulatory vision at the last follow-up examination. The causes were string syndrome (2), cataract (1), keratopathy (2), macular scar (1), and 2 where the reason was unknown. All these patients belonged to the early group. All successfully attached giant tears in the late group achieved ambulatory vision or better, the best even achieving a visual acuity of 1.0 with a contact lens.

In no special field of retinal surgery have the success rates improved so dramatically in recent years as in the treatment of giant tears. As recently as 1982 Federmann wrote that the treatment of giant tears was one of the most difficult challenges in ophthalmology. With silicone oil, operations are easier, and today an uncomplicated giant tear is considered an operation of low to medium grade difficulty and very good prognosis.

#### 4.1.2.3 Posterior Holes

Whereas posterior holes occurred frequently in our patients in combination with complicated retinal detachments with PVR, isolated holes at the posterior eye pole were relatively rare. They constituted a heterogeneous group of eyes with highly variable initial pathologies. This indication group was comprised of eyes with macular holes with or without deep posterior staphyloma, holes in areas of chorioretinal atrophy or conus defects, holes due to localized traction processes (e.g., after uveitis, venous thrombosis, Terson syndrome, endophthalmitis), and posterior holes after blunt trauma or in high myopia with central vitreous traction. As the initial situations were so varied, it is difficult to present a uniform concept, and a comparison with the scientific literature is hardly possible. We therefore confine our detailed discussion to the group of isolated macular holes.

The concepts regarding the therapy of *macular holes* have changed several times in recent years. Our indications for the application of silicone oil in these eyes are accordingly different today from those of 8 years ago.

Macular holes only rarely lead to detachment and so need not be treated prophylactically (Aaberg et al. 1970). They can, however, cause a detachment in highly myopic eyes and occasionally also after blunt trauma. Therapeutic attempts with cryo- or diathermy coagulation of the macular hole, mostly combined with a central buckling explant (Howard and Campbell 1969, Aaberg et al. 1970, Margherio and Schepens 1972, Klöti 1974, Theodossiadis 1974, Siam 1979, Dellaporta 1983), have not proved very satisfactory as the success rates were not very good (Leaver and Cleary 1975), visual acuity was often heavily damaged by coagulation scars (Margherio and Schepens 1972, Klöti 1974), and, moreover, since external manipulations at the posterior pole in these very long eyes were very difficult and fraught with danger. Scleral resection, as proposed by Meyer-Schwickerath (1968), which was supposed to press the retina back on by way of decreased intraocular volume and thereby compression of the vitreous, was also an indirect procedure not directly aimed at the pathology at hand and did not often produce the desired result.

In 1974 Scott proposed to inject silicone oil (without vitrectomy) in front of the retina in eyes with macular holes. He was able to reattach the retina successfully in 32 eyes. At the same time air and gas injections were popularized as well (McLean and Norton 1974, Laqua 1979); McLean was able to reattach four out of six retinas with it.

In 1982 Gonvers and Machemer reported (1982b) that they had succeeded in reattaching six retinas with macular holes by vitrectomy and gas injection without coagulation of the hole. On the basis of their observations they developed the concept that retinal detachments with macular holes are produced by traction of fine, often invisible, vitreous strands and that it is sufficient to remove this traction by vitrectomy to achieve permanent reattachment. Laqua (1985) was able to confirm the 100% success rate with this method with ten uncomplicated macular holes but could, however, repair only one of four eyes that had already been operated on previously.

This experience led to the present basic concept that macular holes should primarily be operated on with gas without coagulation. Only if a redetachment develops or if it becomes apparent intraoperatively that the retina cannot be stretched enough to fill a very deep posterior staphyloma do we apply silicone oil today. When we do, we usually combine it with endolaser or diathermy coagulation to the edges of the hole. The application of cyanoacrylate tissue adhesive to seal macular holes in deep staphylomata (Sheta et al. 1990) is a new concept whose worth remains to be evaluated.

More recently it has become popular to inject expanding gas without vitrectomy in eyes with uncomplicated macular holes (Mester et al. 1983, Kroll et al. 1985, Miyake 1984, Blankenship and Ibanez-Langlois 1987). The simplicity of the procedure is its advantage, and retinas that cannot be reattached with it (Kroll: 6/20; Miyake: 3/18; Blankenship: 7/19) can then be treated by vitrectomy in a second operation. A disadvantage is the very difficult positioning of the patient. This must be done much more accurately with only a small gas bubble than with an eye completely filled with gas. The idea that the gas bubble dissects the vitreous body away from the central retina and thus relieves traction has not been confirmed. Clemens et al. (1986) found ultrasonographically that in all their eyes the vitreous had been compressed in front of the macula instead.

Our results with macular holes show that retinal attachment can almost always be achieved with silicone oil (20/21) and that the postoperative visual acuity is surprisingly good. Nonetheless, since simpler procedures are available for simple repairs, silicone oil should generally not be used as a primary treatment. Our single failure shows that there are very deep posterior staphylomata in which the retina cannot be reattached permanently, not even with silicone oil. For these eyes Ando et al. have taken up the idea of a macular buckling procedure and developed a flexible silicon explant (1988), which they use in such eyes without coagulation. The future will show whether this procedure is suited to treat other complicated macular holes and whether it can entirely substitute for silicone oil in this indication group.

As already mentioned above, the *other posterior holes* in our series represent a heterogeneous group, which as such has found little attention in the literature so far.

In 17 of the 26 eyes in this group we found holes in chorioretinal scars. (see Color Plate 1, Figs. 3a + b). We used silicone oil to tamponade these defects, which are difficult to coagulate, on a long-term basis. In addition we tried to close them with cryotherapy, laser coagulation, or endodiathermy. In 13 of the 17 eyes the retina was finally attached. We have so far, however, removed the silicone oil from only six eyes. We and the patients are very reluctant to remove the oil in such situations, particularly if an only eye is involved. If a hole is not reliably closed, the risk of redetachment is high. It remains to be seen whether attempts to achieve closure of such defects with cyanoacrylate (McCuen et al. 1986, Sheta et al. 1986), fibrin adhesive (Emmerich et al. 1988) or other 'bioadhesives' (Jaffe et al. 1989) will open new possibilities.

The remaining eyes with posterior holes included one with a coloboma of the optic nerve and eight unusual holes in the macular area: three after blunt trauma, one after endophthalmitis, and one after a Fukala procedure with torn out central laser scars. In all of these except two of the three eyes with blunt trauma, we succeeded in attaching the retina. Redetachment developed in the two cases with trauma some time after silicone oil removal. We left the oil in the eye with the coloboma for 3 years; a slight, but controllable secondary glaucoma developed, and visual acuity was stable at 0.05. In all other eyes we were able to remove the silicone oil successfully.

Eyes with posterior holes can be reliably treated with silicone oil. In uncomplicated situations, however, alternative, simpler procedures are available, and at first an attempt at vitrectomy with gas without coagulation is usually justified. In the case of failure, silicone oil with coagulation can then be applied in a second operation.

#### 4.1.2.4 Proliferative Diabetic Retinopathy

Vitreous surgery is accepted and established for the treatment of late complications of PDR. The success rates which can be achieved by vitrectomy alone depend essentially on the initial anatomic situations.

In a comparison Krampitz-Glaas and Laqua (1986) have demonstrated that in 82% of eyes with a simple vitreous hemorrhage without retinal detachment long-term success can be achieved. The success rate declines to 75% if there is extramacular detachment, is reduced further, to 59%, with traction detachment of the macula. Thompson et al. (1986b) calculated the most important negative factors influencing surgical success after vitrectomy in 1007 eyes by logistic regression analysis. The preoperative factors are: vitreous hemorrhage, little or no preceding photocoagulation, traction detachment, retinal holes, active preretinal neovascularization, rubeosis iridis, and cataract. The most important intraoperative factor influencing the prognosis, is the occurrence of iatrogenic defects. The risk of not achieving ambulatory vision postoperatively is, for instance, trebled by traction detachment and even quadrupled by a rhegmatogenous traction detachment existing preoperatively. Iatrogenic defects increase the risk by a factor of 1.76 and rubeosis iridis by 3.1. A completely or partly attached vitreous is by clinical experience an additional, important risk factor which is difficult to measure and was probably not included by Thompson and colleagues in their calculations for this reason.

For the more simple situations, e.g., uncomplicated vitreous hemorrhage, simple traction detachment at the posterior pole without rhegmatogenous component, or active proliferations a simple vitrectomy is all that is needed and will yield good results.

For complicated situations with preexistent or intraoperatively developed retinal defects and active proliferations, the results with vitrectomy and possibly gas are considerably worse. Again comparison of the literature is difficult because of the great number of risk factors involved and their different incidence in the various series. The most important publications on the results of vitrectomy with complicated PDR are listed in Table 15 indicating the risk factors reported. Most series were comprised of a surgically and prognostically very much more favorable group of patients than ours. Michels (1978) and Blankenship and Machemer (1978), for instance, included only 11% and 43%, respectively, of the traction detachments in their series. Aaberg (1979) and Charles (1980) reported solely on eyes with traction detachment and excluded those with vitreous hemorrhage. Although Rice et al. (1983) reported exclusively on traction detachments, they excluded those which had a rhegmatogenous component preoperatively. Thompson and colleagues analyzed their series of 360 eyes with traction detachment with respect to risk factors (1987a + b). Table 15 shows clearly that the success rates worsen as the number of risk factors increases.

The patients with PDR that we operated on with silicone oil also showed a high proportion of risk factors. We used silicone oil in 124 eyes with diabetic traction detachment, most of which also had a preexisting rhegmatogenous component (40 eyes), a necessity for retinotomy and retinectomy, inadvertent smaller iatrogenic defects (44 eyes), with rubeosis iridis (22 eyes), or previous surgery (15 eyes). These patients also had extraordinarily fulminant neovascularizations.

We operated on eyes without these complicating factors – about two thirds of our diabetic patients with vitrectomies – without silicone oil. Often the decision to inject silicone oil was only made intraoperatively, when situations developed which, by experience, could have taken a deleterious course without the use of silicone oil, e.g., when preexisting traction defects were found unexpectedly, when difficult membrane peeling had resulted in multiple iatrogenic holes, or when massive proliferations that could not be separated from the retina necessitated retinectomies (see Color Plate 2, Figs. 2a + 2b).

In comparison with other series operated on without silicone oil, our cohort is therefore probably best compared to the subgroups of Thompson et al. which included eyes with rhegmatogenous detachment or iatrogenic hole formation. The success rates in these groups were 43% and 56%, respectively.

Based on the same criteria and statistical methods applied by these authors, an analysis of our diabetics showed that 66% of them reached at least ambulatory vision at the end of the follow-up period of 18.8 months on average (Thompson et al., 19 months).

So far there have been only a few publications on the use of silicone oil in the treatment of PDR, and most of them use different inclusion criteria or different surgical techniques and are therefore really not comparable with this study. Faulborn (1984) reported on 9 of 16 successfully operated on diabetics, but did not specify how many of those eyes that had a traction detachment were successfully treated. Four further studies (Lean et al. 1982, Gnad et al. 1986, McLeod 1986 and Brourman et al. 1989) reported results that were considerably worse than ours, probably due to the fact that they usually did not remove all proliferative membranes, but instead tried to use the oil to press down a stiff retina. It is well known by now that this approach can lead to fulminant reproliferation. De Corral and Peyman (1986) used the oil in nine diabetics exclusively to prevent a progression of

**Table 15.** Risk factors and visual success rates after vitrectomy for proliferative diabetic retinopathy

| Study(year) | *n* | Rubeosis iridis | Traction detach. | Vitreous hemorrh. | Rhegm. detach. | Iatrog. hole | Visual acuity ≥1/50 |
|---|---|---|---|---|---|---|---|
| | % | % | % | % | % | % | |
| Michels (1978) | 134 | 0 | 11 | 83 | 7 | 4 | 65 |
| Blankenship et al. (1978) | 56 | 13 | 43 | 71 | na | 21 | 50 |
| Aaberg (1979) | 75 | na | 100 | 0 | 0 | 7 | 69 |
| Charles (1980) | 341 | na | 100 | 0 | na | na | 67 |
| Rice et al. (1983) | 204 | 7 | 100 | 41 | 0 | 20 | 59 |
| Thompson et al. (1987a) | 360 | 6 | 100 | na | 0 | 22 | 64 |
| Thompson et al. (1987a) | 79 | 6 | 100 | na | 0 | 100 | 52 |
| Thompson et al. (1987b) | 172 | 6 | 100 | na | 100 | 31 | 56 |
| Thompson et al. (1987b) | 53 | 6 | 100 | na | 100 | 100 | 43 |
| *This series (1990)* | 124 | 18 | 100 | na | 37 | 63 | 66 |

na, not available

rubeosis iridis, McCuen and Rinkoff (1989) limited themselves to eyes that, after preceding vitrectomy, developed a detachment and neovascularizations in the anterior segment. In the series of 106 eyes analyzed by Heimann and colleagues (1989) the results of a subgroup of 91 eyes with traction detachment were not analyzed separately, and the series also included eyes in which proliferative membranes were left undissected. Again, a direct comparison with our results is not possible.

Considering the difficult preoperative anatomic situations, the technical problems at surgery, and the pathologic changes in the inner retina usually present in such severe diabetic retinopathies, our results are encouraging. Comparison with Thompson's figures shows that in the most complicated situations involving PDR with traction detachment the results with silicone oil can be better than those without. Our capabilities are, however, limited by both problems of surgical technique and inherent pathology. The anatomic and functional failures can by and large be attributed to three factors:

1. In one third of the failures we did not succeed in attaching the retina intraoperatively. In seven eyes peripheral traction membranes remained with vitreous attached to them. In two eyes subretinal strands and in another two eyes massive intraoperative hemorrhages with subretinal extension were responsible for failure.
2. Other anatomic failures were the result of heavy fibrotic proliferations mostly at the posterior pole, which often formed characteristic, dense, fibrous preretinal membranes. Reproliferations in eyes with PVR look different, probably due to the fact that they are more of glial than fibrovascular origin (Foos 1978). It has been suggested that the development of this "reparative epiretinal fibrosis" might be favored by a concentration of blood, fibrin, and proliferative factors between the retina and the silicone oil bubble. Such membranes, however, also appear in eyes that were never filled with silicone oil. They are probably the continuation of the fibrovascular proliferative process that necessitated surgery in the first place, possibly stimulated further by retinal trauma during delamination of the membranes (Barry et al. 1985). In view of the advanced pathology in our patients' eyes and the many stimulating factors produced by such traumatizing surgery (blood among others), it is not surprising that such membranes appeared quite frequently. Similar to PVR, there is no conclusive evidence that the development of such membranes is stimulated by the presence of silicone oil.
3. There was a high rate of diabetic retinal and optic atrophies which resulted in progressive loss of vision in a relatively large proportion of the successfully operated on eyes. This was certainly due to preexistent retinal and optic nerve damage caused by the diabetic vasculopathy,

and also frequently occurs in serious cases of PDR in which the eyes are operated on without silicone oil.

*Rubeosis iridis and neovascular glaucoma* are well-documented and dreaded complications after vitrectomy in PDR. Their exact pathogenesis is basically unknown. One theory suggests that removal of the vitreous body enables the diffusion of assumed angiogenic factors into the anterior segment of the eye. Another one assumes that, because of removal of the vitreous body, oxygen can diffuse more easily from the anterior to the posterior segment and that rubeosis is then caused by relatively poor oxygenation of the iris, whereas the better oxygen supply in the posterior segment effects a stabilization of the proliferative retinopathy (Stefánsson et al. 1982). Both these effects would be intensified by lens removal.

The reported incidence of rubeosis iridis after pars plana vitrectomy varies depending on the preoperative pathology and lens status. Klemen et al. (1981) found a postoperative incidence of rubeosis of 9% in vitrectomy eyes with simple vitreous hemorrhage and of 39% in eyes with preretinal membranes and partial or total retinal detachment. If in the context of vitrectomy the lens is extracted, as was commonly done in vitreous surgery in the early years, the rate of newly developed cases of rubeosis iridis can reach 42% overall and 30% following successful operations (Michels 1978). Aaberg (1979) and Krampitz-Glaas and Laqua (1986) with rather mixed cohorts, reported an incidence of new cases of rubeosis of 16% and 17%, respectively. Rice and colleagues (1983) found an incidence of 33% in their patients with traction detachment (45% in aphakic and 18% in phakic eyes). In their cohorts with traction detachment Thompson et al. (1987b) found a 6% incidence of rubeosis iridis preoperatively and a 22%-24% incidence postoperatively. In their subgroup with traction detachment only 38% of the patients with preexisting rubeosis reached ambulatory vision postoperatively, while in the subgroup with a rhegmatogenous component all eyes with preoperative rubeosis ended up blind. Rubeosis iridis as an indicator of a bad anatomic and functional prognosis has already been discussed (p. 95).

When we and others began to fill the eyes of patients who had the most complicated PDRs with silicone oil, we were surprised at the relatively low incidence of rubeosis iridis and neovascular glaucoma in a group of patients in which the worst could be expected. De Juan et al. (1986b) were able to show that the partial oxygen pressure in vitrectomized aphakic eyes is reduced without silicone oil and normal again in eyes filled with silicone oil. They concluded that either the effect demonstrated by Stefánsson is prevented by silicone oil or that silicone oil may inhibit the diffusion of angiogenic substances into the anterior segment and thus have an inhibiting effect on the development of rubeosis iridis and neovascular glaucoma.

In our silicone oil patients we found rubeosis iridis in 16% of the eyes preoperatively; 14% developed in the postoperative period. The preoperative incidence was considerably higher than in all other publications on the subject and may be taken as an indication of the poor preoperative state of the eyes in our series. Considering the advanced pathology, a rate of 14% new cases of iris neovascularizations is surprisingly low. Whereas it is not surprising that our failures had a higher preoperative rate of rubeosis (23%) than the successfully operated on eyes (14%), it is surprising that the rate of newly developed cases is very similar in both groups (successes 15%, failures 13%). We conclude that silicone oil effectively prevents the development of rubeosis iridis in eyes with redetachment. This effect was also described by others (McLeod 1986, Rinkoff et al. 1986).

We can also confirm the observation of Thompson et al. (1987b) that eyes with preoperative rubeosis have a worse prognosis regarding ambulatory vision (41% in this series) than eyes without rubeosis (64%). This is likely to be attributed to the fact that patients with a preoperative rubeosis have a more advanced ischemic retinopathy which eventually results in retinal and optic atrophy, a process silicone oil cannot influence.

In our series, the relatively uncomplicated postoperative clinical course in eyes with rubeosis iridis is remarkable. Four successfully operated on eyes with neovascular glaucoma, all of whom had a rubeosis preoperatively, could be controlled quite quickly with cyclotherapy. A fifth one was stabilized with pilocarpine alone. Of the patients with newly developed rubeosis, only two developed glaucoma: one was successfully treated medically; the other one, who developed glaucoma during a redetachment, normalized spontaneously after retinal reattachment. Whereas we experienced serious problems with high intraocular pressures in five eyes with redetachment, only one of them had to be enucleated for uncontrollable neovascular glaucoma.

Nine cases of secondary glaucoma among the diabetics are difficult to explain. In light of all accompanying circumstances (juvenile diabetics with most massive neovascularizations at the posterior pole), we prefer to think of them as neovascular glaucomas, although we never saw new vessels on the iris. It is conceivable that neovascularizations in the trabecular meshwork can exist subclinically, which then postoperatively led to raised intraocular pressure when surgical trauma and inflammation, perhaps combined with the additional burden of some emulsification, supervene. All of these secondary glaucomas were normalized medically (p. 66).

About 5% – 8% of eyes with advanced PDR develop massive fibrinous exudation postvitrectomy which almost invariably ends in failure and *phthisis* (Sebestyen 1982, Aaberg 1989). The incidence of phthisis in the literature ranges from 9% to 32% after diabetic vitrectomy (Blankenship and

Machemer 1978, Rice and Michels 1980). In our series we did not see the complication of fibrinous exudation as described by Aaberg and only five of the diabetic eyes in our series, all with detached retinas, had some degree of hypotony at the last follow-up examination. None of the patients had painful phthisical changes or visible shrinkage of the eye.

We injected silicone oil into the eyes of 12 diabetics without retinal detachment solely to achieve postoperative *hemostasis*. Two eyes had been given up as inoperable during surgery and the silicone oil was only injected to stabilize an otherwise lost eye. The other instances involved either the only eye (8 patients), with the motive being speedy visual rehabilitation, or young diabetics with fulminant proliferations, in which we injected the silicone oil to avoid postoperative complications such as rubeosis and secondary hemorrhage (two patients), which was considered to be inevitable otherwise (see Color Plate 2, Figs. 1a + b). In all these eyes the retina was attached at the last follow-up examination. With the exception of one eye with retinal and optic atrophy all had a visual acuity of between 1/30 and 0.2. Despite two occurrences of rubeosis none of the eyes developed secondary glaucoma or keratopathy. We were meanwhile able to remove the silicone oil in 7 of these latter 10 eyes without any problems. This uncomplicated course certainly justified this otherwise unusual indication for silicone oil.

Silicone oil in PDR thus serves several purposes:

1. We have used it primarily as a *tamponade* in complicated cases, in eyes with multiple or extensive retinal defects, which, by experience, we have found to have a poor prognosis without oil. Although the development of preretinal proliferations, which often lead to redetachment, are of great concern to us and are perhaps stimulated by the presence of the oil, the anatomic success rate in these desolate situations is certainly better with silicone oil than it would be without.
2. The *hemostatic effect* of silicone oil is of great advantage. It allows fast visual rehabilitation, laser treatment when needed, and a good control over the retinal situation.
3. Silicone oil inhibits the development of *rubeosis iridis* even though it cannot always prevent it. In eyes with preexisting rubeosis this rarely progresses, and the incidence of severe neovascular glaucoma is obviously greatly reduced.
4. Silicone oil can often prevent the development of painful *phthisis*. Even in blind eyes silicone oil still has a stabilizing effect, which on its own may already be of advantage considering the often limited life expectancy of these severely affected diabetics.

Silicone oil cannot prevent progressive retinal and optic atrophy despite successful surgery. Thus the long-term prospect for the preservation of ambulatory vision unfortunately amounts to only 60%.

#### 4.1.2.5 Perforating Injuries

The incidence of severe ocular injuries has declined steadily due to higher awareness of safety and ever improving preventive measures. To the same extent, however, the surgical possibilities have expanded in recent years so that the proportion of patients with perforating injuries out of the total number of patients has remained more or less stable with time.

The group of eyes with perforating injuries was extraordinarily heterogeneous. The prognosis was determined by a great number of factors differing from eye to eye. These were among others:

1. *Type of injury*: blunt or sharp trauma, severity of the contusion force, sharp or blunt foreign body, simple or double perforation, magnetic or amagnetic foreign body, bacterial contamination, size of the wound
2. *Tissues concerned*: aniridia, lens involvement, ciliary body, vitreous, retinal or choroidal injury, massive choroidal detachment, vitreous hemorrhage
3. *Site of injury*: e.g., involvement of the vitreous base (causing increased proliferation), direct injury of the macula (hardly any surgical possibilities)
4. *Surgical care*: timing of primary and secondary care, time and method of foreign body removal, prophylactic encircling band, early vitrectomy

The greatest problem with injuries of the posterior eye segment is the ensuing PVR which is virtually inevitable. In principle it is the same process as already described above for PVR; its course, however, is often considerably more fulminant. The objective of attending to severe injuries therefore is to prevent, or at least control, this proliferative process.

The surgical objectives of vitrectomy of perforating injuries are manifold. They include: the extraction of intraocular foreign bodies that cannot be removed with a magnet; the removal of blood from the vitreous cavity, which has a considerable share in stimulation of the proliferative process (Benson and Machemer 1976, Hutton and Fuller 1984); and that of the vitreous body itself, which offers a scaffold for the growth of proliferative cells and probably contains additional factors stimulating proliferation. Vitrectomy, furthermore, allows the removal of proliferative membranes that have already developed, relief of retinal traction, and, by improving the view of the fundus, closure of retinal defects by conventional retinal surgery (for an exemplary case see Color Plate 2, Figs. 3a + b).

The correct timing for vitrectomy of eyes after perforating trauma is crucial; the decision when to intervene, however, is a very difficult one to make. There are a great number of studies showing conclusively that a PVR can be best prevented if surgical intervention takes place as early as possible (Faulborn and Topping 1978, Abrams et al. 1979, Heimann et al. 1979, Coleman 1982, Chen 1983), but the danger of massive intraoperative hemorrhages is extremely high within the first 10 days after an injury, and a vitrectomy is technically very difficult before vitreous detachment has occurred, usually by about two weeks. Therefore, most ophthalmic surgeons recommend that initially only primary wound closure and foreign body removal should be performed, and vitreous surgery should be delayed until 10 – 14 days after the injury. We know though that by that time PVR has already developed in many eyes. Thus recent strategies aim at performing a vitrectomy, at least in the most seriously injured eyes, at once or at least within 3 days after the injury (Coleman 1982). Should massive hemorrhages occur, they can be controlled intraoperatively by silicone oil as an intraocular tamponade. Skorpik et al. (1987) and Lemmen and Heimann (1988a) were able to achieve surprising success with this approach in some very badly injured eyes with otherwise desolate prognoses. The argumentation in favor of an early surgical intervention is supported additionally by animal experiments (Lemmen et al. 1988b) showing that early silicone oil injection after experimental perforating injuries can very effectively prevent the occurrence of detachment and PVR, which otherwise would be practically unavoidable.

Consequently, silicone oil is used for the treatment of perforating injuries in four basic situations: (1) when a proliferative vitreoretinopathy has already set in, (2) as a primary injection to prevent PVR in eyes at high risk, (3) as an effective tamponade of large retinal defects, e.g., large retinectomies for the relief of retinal incarceration in scleral wounds (Han et al. 1988), and (4) for intraoperative or postoperative hemostasis in eyes with a high tendency to hemorrhage.

Almost without exception our 61 patients with perforating injuries were operated on some days or weeks after injury. Only five eyes still had intraocular foreign bodies at the time of the silicone oil operation, in one eye three amagnetic metal splinters were found intraretinally. All eyes already had a retinal detachment, and 47 eyes already had an overt PVR. There were 38 eyes that were operated on before; in 28 of them this had already been aimed at reattaching a detached retina. Some 12 eyes had subretinal strands; in 13 eyes the retina was incarcerated at the site of impact or rupture and had to be freed by retinectomy. This illustrates that our cases can be regarded as particularly complicated. Due to the highly variable clinical features a comparison of our results with those of other authors with and without silicone oil (Cinotti and Maltzman 1975, Faulborn et al. 1976, Heimann et al.1978, Brinton et al. 1982, Lemmen et al. 1984, Lemmen and Heimann 1988a, Antoszyk et al. 1989, Skorpik et al. 1989) is not reasonable.

Considering the severity of the initial pathologies, a 61% anatomic success rate 2 years after surgery must, at the moment, be regarded as the limit of what can be done. If there was a possibility of preventing or checking reproliferation medically (p. 3), further improvements would be conceivable. These successes were, however, associated with a rather high incidence of complications: 6 of the 11 enucleated eyes in our series had perforating injuries, 2 eyes with trauma had a clinically distinct phthisis, and 5 eyes had not visibly shrunk, but had persistent pressures below 5 mm Hg. With 13% this indication group had the highest incidence of newly developed keratopathies. Only the rate of secondary glaucoma was low; this however might possibly be explained by the fact that some potential glaucomas were masked by hypofunction of the ciliary body.

Our experience in the last years has shown that many eyes with perforating injuries in which serious complications have already occurred can still be saved with silicone oil surgery. The oil in this context basically fulfills the same functions as in PVR: tamponading multiple or large retinal defects and modifying membrane growth to prevent inoperable situations. Nonetheless as we have already shown with giant tears, silicone oil can evidently prevent or at least check the development of PVR only if it is applied early enough. This certainly holds true for perforating trauma as well. The present trend moves towards surgery as early as possible. We recently took this approach in a few patients, performing a vitrectomy before PVR developed, and filling high risk eyes with silicone oil early, and we were quite satisfied with the results. There is therefore every reason to believe that the success rates after serious injuries can be further improved.

#### 4.1.2.6 Other Indications

Our experience with the eyes classified among "other indications" was rather varied.

Only in one eye with an *acute retinal necrosis* were we able to reattach the retina permanently, preserving good visual acuity (0.4) after performing a 360° retinectomy. This patient has already been reported on (Lucke et al. 1988). We did manage to reattach a second retina with acute retinal necrosis but the eye had no function as a result of optic nerve atrophy. In this patient and in a third one surgery came too late; the disease had progressed too far. We lost a fourth eye with acute retinal necrosis in spite of intensive therapy and early vitrectomy before the onset of retinal detachment. Future studies will show whether the generally poor prognosis can be improved upon possibly with more intensive intravitreal virostatic therapy (Blumenkranz et al. 1986), perhaps combined with extensive laser coagulation (Sternberg et al. 1988) and early long-term tamponade with gas or silicone oil (Blumenkranz et al. 1988, Anand and Fisher 1988).

In two eyes with *Eales' disease* we succeeded initially at reattaching the retina. In one eye, however, redetachment occurred 15 months after we removed the oil. Revision surgery was only partially successful. In the second eye the retina was, in fact, attached, but there was complete atrophy of the optic nerve and a neovascular glaucoma. No conclusions can be drawn from the experiences with these two eyes, but it seems to us that eyes with both Eales' disease and traction detachment have an extremely poor prognosis.

Our experience with two eyes with *uveitis* and advanced traction detachment was similar. In one eye the retina was attached, but visual acuity, due to optic nerve atrophy, was reduced to hand movement. The same as with Eales' disease can be said here. The prognosis in such cases is basically poor, and the use of silicone oil must be carefully considered in each situation.

In one eye with *Coats' disease*, hypotony, rubeosis iridis, and exudative detachment we injected the silicone oil basically only to "stabilize" the eye. Almost 2 years later, the exudative neovascular process in the retinal periphery had regressed, the retina was attached, the pressure had slowly risen to 9 mm Hg, and visual acuity remained stable at 0.05. A keratopathy caused by silicone oil prolapse during the period of hypotony had regressing after the eye began to normalize its pressure and the silicone was no longer in contact with the cornea. Without silicone oil this only eye would certainly have been blind. Uncertainty must remain as to whether we prevented blindness or simply postponed it. In operations such as this one every surgical action and particularly the use of silicone oil must be critically evaluated. Silicone oil surgery is certainly only justified in uniocular patients and even then only if the patient has decided on surgery in full awareness of the poor long-term prognosis.

In one eye with massive subretinal hemorrhage due to *disciform macular degeneration* we succeeded in removing the blood via a large circumferential peripheral retinotomy, improving visual acuity temporarily to 0.05. Unfortunately the patient never returned for follow-up, and we know from her ophthalmologist that the retina redetached. A massive PVR probably developed in the postoperative course, a complication that has been observed by other authors after such an operation too (C.Eckardt, J.Petersen, personal communication). The surgical removal of subretinal hemorrhage and exudative tissue in this disease, as described by Živojnović (1987), cannot restore visual acuity, but may sometimes preserve some peripheral field of vision. Although age-related macular degeneration is a frequent affliction, serious forms such as this one are fortunately rare. The prognosis in such cases is very poor, but an attempt at surgery particularly in the only eye is sometimes certainly justified.

In one eye with *optic-nerve and choroidal coloboma* we were able to reattach the retina with silicone oil. Visual acuity of this only eye was, in fact, only counting fingers, but the field of vision was good, the postoperative course free of complications, and the patient was very satisfied. Whether retinal detachments with coloboma of the optic nerve are caused by retinal holes in the coloboma, an exudative process, or even subretinal cerebrospinal fluid is still not known (Schatz and McDonald 1988). In our patient the retina had spontaneously reattached permanently after vitrectomy and silicone oil injection. This speaks for a rhegmatogenous pathogenesis even though at no time were we able to identify a retinal break.

## 4.1.3 Complications

### 4.1.3.1 Intraoperative Complications

Intraoperative complications caused by silicone oil are rare and can generally be avoided by good surgical technique. The fact that 12 of our 13 subretinal silicone oil infusions were found among our first 100 operations is a clear indication that this complication, formerly so much dreaded, is avoidable. Complete freedom of retinal traction is an absolute prerequisite for silicone oil injection. The oil should never be injected with the objective of pressing the retina down. Furthermore, it is very helpful to have a good and wide view of the fundus during oil injection – indirect ophthalmoscopy and oil-fluid exchange make this much easier.

During silicone oil injection, massive hypertony can also be avoided with good surgical technique, keeping the point of the flute needle, under direct observation, always safely in the liquid phase and constantly palpating the intraocular pressure with one finger towards the end of the injection process. Again with careful surgical technique silicone oil passage into the anterior chamber intraoperatively can be avoided. If this nevertheless does happen, the oil can be removed from the anterior chamber by relatively simple means.

#### 4.1.3.2 Cataract

It is widely accepted that the development of a cataract is practically unavoidable when silicone oil is used. Although cataract rates of about 80% are reported in the literature (Dimopoulos and Heimann 1986, Grey and Leaver 1977, Živojnović et al. 1981), it is only a question of the length of follow-up for this rate to reach 100%.

The cause of cataract formation is unclear. While lens epithelium is known to occasionally undergo profound changes in eyes with complicated retinal detachments even in the absence of silicone oil (Scott 1982) cataracts that were removed from eyes treated with silicone oil and examined histologically did not show any unusual characteristics (Haut et al. 1980a). Silicone oil vacuoles in the lens itself have never been found, only once was a silicone oil vacuole on the lens capsule described. General opinion among silicone oil surgeons holds that cataract formation is therefore more a mechanical effect than a toxic one: the silicone oil bubble prevents the diffusion of metabolically vital substances to the lens. This leads to an early opacification of the posterior cortex and, later on, to the development of nuclear sclerosis. We observed a lens that was only partially opacified in an eye where only that part of the lens was in contact with silicone oil (see Color Plate 3, Figs. 3a + b).

A mechanical cause of cataract formation explains why it also occurs when the vitreous cavity is filled with long-acting gases (A.Lincoff et al. 1983; H.Lincoff et al. 1983). Such a disturbance of the natural diffusion process is probably also responsible for the lens being damaged even after simple vitrectomy. In a series of 90 patients with vitrectomy for macular pucker, Michels (1984) found 34% with postoperative cataract. De Bustros et al. (1988) reported on 63% newly developed or progressive nuclear scleroses after pucker surgery.

Eckardt (1986) found that in rabbit eyes irreversible damage to the lens developed as early as 1-2 weeks after silicone oil injection. Although this cannot necessarily be applied to human lenses, attempts to avoid cataract formation by early removal of the silicone oil as a matter of routine have failed. Gonvers (1985) removed the oil after 6 weeks as a rule, but then found out that 61% of the lenses, having remained clear up till then, became opaque later on. Early removal of silicone oil does not really make sense as long-term tamponade is precisely the specific advantage of silicone oil over intraocular gases.

In some diabetics cataract formation is apparently delayed. Here and in some other eyes not in need of long-term tamponade, we therefore tried to avoid a cataract by early silicone oil removal. Although this was only successful in 4 of 29 eyes, this procedure can be tried in selected cases if the patient is aware of the fact that this may eventually necessitate an additional operation.

With every form of long-term tamponade eventual lens extraction is practically unavoidable. For reasons of surgical technique a primary lens extraction is usually performed in gas surgery. Many silicone oil surgeons also remove the lens in the primary procedure, in expectation of cataract and assuming that the oil will be retained for a long time. In these situations the question of late cataract formation is of course irrelevant. We, however, prefer to preserve the lens in the primary procedure if possible since it affords good protection for the anterior segment. We then generally remove the lens secondarily, together with the silicone oil. Later we tried to implant intraocular lenses in selected patients.

#### 4.1.3.3 Emulsification

The term "emulsification" has come into general usage for a process in which small, stable, silicone droplets separate from the large intravitreal silicone bubble and spread into ocular tissues. They can typically be found in the anterior chamber angle (at 12 o'clock), on the iris surface, between the zonular fibers, in front of the ciliary body, and preretinally in the upper half of the fundus.

The causes of this droplet formation have not been fully explained yet. Present concepts comprise three mechanisms:

1. Bipolar molecules in the eye, so-called emulsifiers (e.g., phospholipids), might stabilize mechanically shorn off parts of the silicone bubble in the eye and prevent the return of these small droplets into the main bubble. Theoretical considerations, stating that oils of higher viscosity and such with a smaller proportion of short molecular chains tend to emulsify to a lesser degree, were confirmed by Crisp et al. (1987) in a laboratory model with benzalkonium chloride as the emulsifying agent.
2. According to Kreiner (1987) the emulsification droplets might be the result of vaporization of volatile components of silicone oil. The oil then diffuses in the gaseous state to a place of lower temperature and there condenses again forming droplets. Only shorter molecular chains would be capable of undergoing this process. Thus, as proposed by Crisp, purified oils should emulsify to a lesser degree than unpurified ones.
3. Macrophages might have a share in the process of emulsification. Intraperitoneally injected silicone oil is phagocytozed by macrophages (Failer et al. 1984, Champion et al. 1987). Similarly macrophages with large vacuoles can be found in enucleated eyes with silicone oil (Rentsch et al. 1977, Leaver et al. 1979b). Rentsch concluded that these macrophages might migrate into the tissue and perish there leaving free silicone oil droplets. Failer (1984) showed that there was less phago-

cytosis in highly viscous oils (60 000 – 100 000 cps) than in low viscosity oils.

All three concepts therefore lead to the conclusion that highly purified and highly viscous silicone oils should show less of a tendency towards emulsification. Riedel et al. (1990), in their cohort of eyes operated on with silicone oil OP5000 exclusively, found an incidence of overt emulsification of only 0,7%. Petersen and Ritzau-Tondrow (1988a) found the rate of glaucoma due to emulsification to be significantly higher in eyes operated on with purified oil of a viscosity of 1000 cps compared to eyes operated on with a similar oil of 5000 cps. We can also confirm these theoretical considerations clinically although our data are insufficient to prove these observations statistically. We have in fact seen emulsification, "inverse hypopion" formation, and emulsification glaucoma with both the unpurified silicone oil SF96 and with the purified OP5000, but these phenomena have become rare since introduction of the purified oil of higher viscosity and only very occasionally do they constitute a clinical problem. We recently observed a patient in whom we could detect no overt emulsification 15 months after surgery of his right eye with silicone oil OP5000, whereas there was an "inverse hypopion"in his left eye 12 months after silicone surgery of his left eye with silicone oil OP1000 performed elsewhere (see Color Plate 4, Figs 3a + b). In eyes with clinically significant emulsification and raised intraocular pressure we were usually able to normalize the pressure on a long-term basis by removing the silicone oil.

The degree of emulsification differs widely from patient to patient. Some eyes have only a few droplets in the upper chamber angle after many years of silicone oil filling, whereas others develop massive emulsification with the formation of an "inverse hypopion" within a few months. It can be speculated that different concentrations of various biological emulsifiers in the aqueous might be responsible for this variability.

The problem of emulsification is specific to silicone oil; with gas comparable problems, of course, do not exist. In principle emulsification occurs to some degree in all oil treated eyes, but evidently causes problems only in a few. Emulsification as such could be accepted if it was not associated with glaucoma.

#### 4.1.3.4 Glaucoma

Until recently the development of glaucoma after silicone oil surgery was regarded as being causally related to the oil itself. This was partly based on older studies, in which silicone oil particles and macrophages were found in the trabecular meshwork (Ni et al. 1983, Rentsch 1977), and which thereby demonstrated a possible mechanism for "silicone oil glaucoma", namely, an overloading of the trabecular meshwork with silicone oil droplets.

Our results show, however, that there are definitely several causes for postoperatively raised intraocular pressure and glaucoma. The analysis of these problems is difficult: In such a heterogeneous group of patients statistical evaluation can only point out trends and is of very limited value. Analysis of each single affected eye proved to be much more useful for gaining additional information about these special glaucoma problems.

Raised intraocular pressures could be divided into two groups: temporary and persisting. This division is artificial and can only provide a limited picture, as a "persistent glaucoma" had to be defined as a glaucoma existing at the last follow-up examination. It is possible that some of these will have to be assigned to the temporary group in the future, if the pressures should later decrease. As opposed to the classical chronic, open-angle glaucoma many of the raised intraocular pressures in the temporary group of patients were spontaneously reversible and therefore better defined as "temporary postoperative pressure increases".

Furthermore, it is important to keep in mind that some of these eyes probably had an increased outflow resistance preoperatively, which was masked by the hypotony caused by retinal detachment, and were therefore not registered as having preexisting glaucoma. Conversely, some eyes may not be included in the glaucoma statistics because a postoperatively increased outflow resistance was neutralized by hypofunction of the ciliary body.

The *temporary pressure increases* could be attributed to angle- and pupillary-block situations, chamber angle pathology, emulsification, and inflammation (p. 63). A clear separation of those pressure increases related to silicone oil from those not related to it was only partly possible.

Pressure increases through angle-block or emulsification can be attributed directly to silicone oil. The prolapse of silicone oil into the anterior chamber and mechanical angle-blocks have become avoidable or at least treatable since the introduction of the inferior basal iridectomy by Ando. It should be expected that with such iridectomies angle-blocks could be avoided altogether and with them synechia formation in the chamber angle and, consequently, some cases of persisting glaucoma. This connection could, however, not be confirmed statistically.

Clinically recognizable emulsification in the sense of an "inverse hypopion" (see Color Plate 4, Fig. 3a), which is actually regarded as the typical cause of a silicone oil glaucoma, was the cause of temporary pressure increases in only three eyes. In all three, the pressure was permanently normalized by immediately removing the oil. The other eyes with variable clinical emulsification, in which the pressures were also normalized by silicone oil removal, were also assigned to this group of "emulsification glaucoma" although we were not able to prove the pathogenesis.

Formation of peripheral anterior synechia, hemorrhage, and inflammatory reactions must be evaluated as causes of increased intraocular pressure that are not connected to silicone oil directly. Protracted inflammatory states sometimes with fibrin formation are frequent after such extensive surgery even without silicone oil, and these eyes need local cortisone therapy often for a long period of time. To date we have not observed unusually strong inflammatory reactions with hypopion formation as did Johnson et al. (1989) in two eyes immediately after silicone oil surgery and which was attributed primarily to an impurity in the oil. Whether silicone oil supports chronic inflammation remains controversial.

Some 11% of the eyes successfully operated on had newly developed *persisting secondary glaucoma* after 22 months on average. In most of them we found an anatomic substrate for the increased pressure. The clinical situations and the possible causes and risk factors are described in detail on pp. 63 – 65.

The picture found is decidedly mixed. The most important factors favoring the development of secondary glaucoma are neovascularization, peripheral anterior synechiae, emulsification, chronic inflammation, glaucoma of the other eye, high myopia, and blunt trauma. In many eyes several of the factors mentioned will play a part; silicone oil emulsification as the only recognizable cause was found in only a very small proportion of patients.

The course of these secondary glaucomas was surprisingly free of complications. We saw only two patients with glaucomatous cupping of the optic disc, and in no patient was a fistulating procedure needed. Most glaucomas could be well controlled by medical therapy alone. When emulsification played an important part, the pressures mostly reverted to normal immediately after silicone oil removal. Occasionally it took a few weeks until glaucoma medication could be discontinued, and in one patient we had to rinse out the remaining droplets in an additional small operation.

A comparison between silicone oil surgery and vitrectomy and gas with respect to glaucoma is difficult and can only be made within individual indication groups. Reports on secondary glaucoma after vitrectomy *without* silicone oil restrict themselves almost without exception to neovascular glaucoma in diabetics; the reported incidence was 10%-21% (Blankenship and Machemer 1978, Krampitz-Glaas and Laqua 1986). The rate of glaucoma after surgery *with* silicone oil varies in the literature from 11% to 22% (Ando 1987, Beekhuis et al. 1985, Chan and Okun 1986, Dimopoulos and Heimann 1986, Haut et al. 1980, Heimann and Dimopoulos 1984a, Leaver et al. 1979a, Sell et al. 1987, Federman and Schubert 1988). It is remarkable in these reports that diabetics and nondiabetics were affected to approximately the same extent (diabetics: 12%; nondiabetics: 8%).

The incidence of glaucoma in diabetics after silicone oil surgery therefore was not any higher than after simple vitrectomy; it was actually probably even lower considering the advanced pathologies in our series. A comparison of glaucoma rates with and without silicone oil in patients with PVR or other indications is unfortunately not possible, however, since the glaucoma problem has been studied in much more detail in silicone oil surgery than in surgery with gas. As a matter of fact, in the four largest series published reporting on the results of PVR and gas surgery (Jalkh et al. 1984, Ho and McMeel 1985, Sternberg and Machemer 1985, Fisher et al. 1988) glaucoma problems are not mentioned at all. It is hard to believe that not one of the 633 cases reported on in these publications ever had a glaucoma.

Our analysis shows, that secondary glaucoma after silicone oil surgery was caused by a great variety of factors. Predisposing factors, such as myopia and diabetes, secondary changes caused by the underlying disease, and surgical trauma, probably played a far bigger role in the pathogenesis than overloading of the trabecular meshwork by emulsification. Emulsification was probably an important contributing factor in predisposed eyes. This, however, could normally be reversed by silicone oil removal. Our figures show that pure "silicone oil glaucoma" was rare, but in the future more attention must be paid to the problem of emulsification in order to limit this factor as much as possible. In principle the problem of glaucoma in silicone oil surgery can probably not be eliminated entirely. Although the glaucomas in our patients were altogether well controllable, they represented the potentially most worrisome complication with an undetermined long-term set of problems.

#### 4.1.3.5 Keratopathy

The most dreaded complication in the early phase of silicone oil surgery was keratopathy, and the published incidences of keratopathy varied between 5.5% and 32% (Leaver et al. 1979a, Haut et al. 1980a, Dimopoulos and Heimann 1986, Heimann and Dimopoulos 1984a, Cox et al. 1986, Riedel et al. 1990). The situation has improved profoundly in the last few years due to the introduction of the inferior basal iridectomy by Ando and due to a better understanding of the causes and prevention; thus an analysis of keratopathy rates is appropriate, especially in the late group.

Clinically and morphologically keratopathies after silicone oil surgery can be divided into two different forms (Lemmen et al. 1987) and occur alone or in combination: *Bullous keratopathies* are the manifestation of massive damage to and numerical reduction of corneal endothelial cells. (see Color Plate 4, Fig. 2b). This process results in edema of the corneal epithelium and in a severe reduction of visual acuity and occurs in many situations in ophthalmology, for instance after cataract surgery.

Reductions of the endothelial cell density have also been described after simple vitrectomy – Friberg (1984) found a 12.6% decrease of endothelial cells after vitrectomy in aphakic eyes. A thinning-out of the endothelium also occurs after injection of gas into the anterior chamber, the severity being dependent on the duration of gas filling (van Horn et al. 1972, Olson 1980, Foulks et al. 1987). Chung and colleagues (1988) found a 2.8% incidence of bullous keratopathy in a series of 428 pars plana vitrectomies without application of silicone oil.

If silicone oil is filled into the anterior chamber of rabbit and cat eyes, a dramatic loss of endothelial cells occurs in the area of permanent contact between silicone oil and endothelium after only a few days. In rabbits Sternberg found a drop of about 60% and in cats of about 40%. In rabbits this loss was reversible after silicone oil removal, not so with cats (Lemmen et al. 1985). Karel and colleagues (1986) examined 22 human eyes with the endothelial microscope after silicone oil surgery. They did not find any changes in endothelial cell count as long as the silicone oil remained behind the pupillary plane. In four eyes with silicone oil prolapse into the anterior chamber with endothelial contact they described a decrease in the density of endothelial cells to 37% of the initial value after 2-3 months and to 16% after 6-12 months.

Endothelial decompensation does not become clinically manifest as long as the silicone oil lines the endothelium and thus prevents edema of the cornea. In such eyes a bullous keratopathy becomes manifest only on the day after silicone oil removal (see Color Plate 4, Figs. 2a + b).

Keratopathies can only be reliably avoided if the silicone oil is effectively prevented from prolapsing into the anterior chamber. The damage caused by silicone oil is, however, not necessarily quite as dramatic as could be expected from Karel's study. Gao and colleagues (1989) found extremely variable reactions of the endothelium to long-term contact with silicone oil. We also saw several patients who did not suffer from endothelial decompensation although the anterior chamber had been filled with silicone oil for many weeks, in one patient even for 8 months.

*Band keratopathy* is caused by long-term contact between silicone oil and corneal endothelium. After some months the cornea becomes opaque in a horizontal band corresponding to the palpebral fissure (see Color Plate 4, Fig. 2a). Brodrick (1978) was able to prove histologically that the opacities are caused by the deposition of calcium phosphate in Bowman's membrane.

Band keratopathies occur frequently outside ophthalmic surgery with manifold ocular and systemic causes. In conjunction with ocular surgery they generally occur in hypotonic, phthisical eyes and in eyes with secondary ischemia of the anterior segment (Grossniklaus et al. 1986), e.g., after string syndrome, extensive muscle surgery and extensive scleral resections. It is assumed that silicone-related band keratopathy is the consequence of inhibition of diffusion through the anterior chamber, which effects an increase of pH in that part of the cornea that is in contact with the atmosphere, i.e. in the palpebral fissure. This secondarily leads to the deposition of calcium phosphate crystals (O'Connor 1969).

In contrast to bullous keratopathies, band keratopathies are reversible and can be considered as clinically relatively benign as they do not necessarily lead to a significant reduction in visual acuity. If necessary, the crystals can be dissolved out of Bowman's membrane with EDTA after epithelial abrasion. They recur, however, if the oil is not removed from the anterior chamber. A band keratopathy can also disappear spontaneously when the oil is finally removed (personal observations).

For the sake of this study, we have considered both forms of keratopathy as potentially caused by silicone oil and, on the whole, not differentiated them any further. Since they cause a common problem, they are discussed together.

In our series the rate of newly developed keratopathies in successfully operated on eyes could be lowered from 11% in the early group to 5% in the late group. The difference is mainly explained by the fact that in the early group the lack of an inferior iridectomy was probably responsible for a band keratopathy in seven eyes. Although we saw quite a few instances of silicone oil prolapse in the late group, since the inferior iridectomies closed up quite frequently, no new keratopathies developed as a consequence since the prolapse was invariably treated immediately.

The remaining keratopathies (Fig. 25) were virtually unavoidable, and it will not be possible to lower the keratopathy rate to zero in a series of such complicated pathologies. Some keratopathies existed already preoperatively; the remaining ones developed as a result of anterior segment trauma or silicone oil prolapse due to hypotony or iris coloboma. String syndrome or glaucoma were rarer causes of keratopathy in our series.

In eyes with redetachment, band keratopathies were more frequent (24% keratopathies after 2 years) due to the the silicone oil being pushed forward by retinal redetachment, the ensuing hypotony, and other factors. Nevertheless, these eyes remained free of complications for surprisingly long periods of time; So far only three eyes had to be enucleated because of a keratopathy.

Keratopathies caused by silicone oil nowadays only occur in eyes in which silicone contact with the corneal endothelium is unavoidable. These are basically reduced to eyes with chronic hypotony or large defects of the iris diaphragm. By the introduction of the inferior iridectomy and because of a better understanding of the degree of filling and the dynamics of the silicone oil bubble, we can avoid long-lasting silicone oil prolapse in the vast majority of eyes. Even in those hypotonic eyes in which a keratopathy has to be accepted, we can, through EDTA abrasion, preserve ambulatory vision, often for a long time. If the pressure normalizes on a long-term basis, the oil can be removed, and, if necessary, a penetrating keratoplasty performed. In the late group this has, however, not been necessary so far. Keratopathy was the cause of vision below ambulatory level in only two eyes in the late group. One eye had a bullous keratopathy already present before the silicone oil procedure, and the other eye had developed a bullous keratopathy after a revision with gas, the eighth operation that had to be performed on that eye. The danger of a possible keratopathy is nowadays no longer a contraindication to the use of silicone oil.

#### 4.1.3.6 Other Complications

*Endophthalmitis* is actually not a complication of silicone oil, as the oil used is sterile. The incidence of endophthalmitis after vitrectomy in the literature ranges from 1:250 to 1:500 (May and Peyman 1976, Blankenship 1977) and should be in about the same range after silicone oil surgery. Živojnović (1987) reported on four cases from more than 1000 silicone oil procedures. We have seen only one case in well over 1000 silicone oil operations.

In eyes filled with silicone oil endophthalmitis takes such an unusual form that this complication should be mentioned, particularly as we have seen a patient who developed an endophthalmitis after perforating injury.

In a similar case Chong and colleagues (1986) pointed out the unusual characteristics of an endophthalmitis in eyes filled with silicone oil. Due to the inert silicon bubble, the anterior segment is relatively protected from the inflammatory process, and the infection is restricted to the immediate retinal vicinity for a long time. As a result of this "compartmentalization" the anterior segment remains relatively uninvolved. Moreover the view through the silicone oil remains clear so that it is difficult to make a diagnosis. Severe pain and the development of a whitish preretinal membrane are characteristic features. The diagnosis of an endophthalmitis must be considered in such an unusual situation. The features of our case support this concept of compartmentalization.

*Scleral fistula* formation is rare and can mostly be attributed to localized atrophy of the sclera in the sclerotomy area after multiple vitrectomies. It can be avoided by good surgical techniques and is not a complication peculiar to silicone oil surgery. A detailed discussion is not necessary.

*Hypotonies* after silicone oil injection are a consequence of disease-related hypofunction of the ciliary body and cannot be directly attributed to silicone oil either. On the contrary, in individual cases silicone oil is used to stabilize eyes with hypotony, and, at least in PDR the frequency of hypotony after silicone oil surgery was lower than that after simple vitrectomy (p. 100). The importance of hypotony after silicone oil surgery lies in the fact that the development of keratopathy can practically not be avoided in affected eyes. This aspect has been discussed above.

### 4.1.4 Retinal Toxicity

Many authors have expressed the opinion that silicone oil has a toxic effect on the retina (Lee et al. 1969, Mukai et al. 1972+1975, Cockerham et al. 1969, Kanski and Daniel 1973, Sugar & Okamura 1976, Manschot 1978, Alexandridis & Daniel 1981, Ni et al. 1983, Gonvers et al. 1986, Jalkh et al. 1986, Kroll et al. 1988a). They largely refer to information of the 1960s and 1970s, but most of them do not rate the problem high enough to not use silicone oil. As a result of more recent studies and clinical observations other authors have doubted this assumption (Okun 1968, Scott 1977, Haut 1980c, Deutmann et al. 1980, Ober et al. 1983, Foerster et a. 1985, Meredith et al. 1985, Chan and Okun 1986, Lucke et al. 1987, Bornfeld et al. 1987, Kellner et al. 1988). The fact that this question evokes controversy among silicone oil surgeons even today is an indication of how difficult it is to prove or disprove this assumption. To debate this central question of silicone oil surgery, we should like to discuss the histological, chemical and electrophysiological studies published and try to relate our functional results to them.

#### 4.1.4.1 Histology

After the initial experiments by Stone (1958) on rabbit eyes, demonstrating a good ocular tolerance to silicone oil, Armaly (1962 a + b) tested the intraocular tolerance of small amounts of silicone oil (Dow Chemical 200) in the anterior chamber and in the vitreous cavity in rabbits, cats, and owl monkeys. The silicone oil was tolerated without signs of inflammation by all animals for 18 months and histologically no indication of tissue reaction, cellular infiltration, or giant cell reaction, and no pathological changes in the cornea, trabecular meshwork, or retina were found. The electroretinograms in the owl monkeys were also normal. Cibis (1962), Levine and Ellis (1963), and Höpping (1964) carried out rabbit experiments confirming these results.

The controversy about the alleged toxicity of silicone oil was then initiated by an experimental investigation on rabbits and owl monkeys by Lee and colleagues (1969), who found considerable changes in the retina histologically after only 2 days of silicone oil filling. The authors demonstrated swelling and vacuolation of the inner nerve fiber layer as well as vacuoles and degenerative changes in the ganglion cells and photoreceptors. These eyes also had extinguished or reduced electroretinograms. The authors pointed out pathological intercellular gaps between Müller cells, through which they presumed the silicone oil might have penetrated the lamina interna. Similar gaps were recently found by Durlu et al. (1990), but there was no evidence suggestive of intraretinal penetration of silicone particles. Further experimental investigations were made by the same group (Mukai 1972 and Mukai 1975), in which, with histochemical methods, massive changes in the enzymatic composition in the inner retinal layers and so-called silicone-lipid complexes between Müller cells were demonstrated. Jalkh et al. (1986) from the same institution, then published a fundus photograph of an eye in which intraretinal silicone oil particles were supposed to be visible. The conclusion was that "silicone oil retinopathy" must become manifest after 5 years at the latest (Ni et al. 1983). Considering the massive changes they had found in the owl monkeys, it is surprising that they did not expect it much sooner.

Other groups were not able to confirm these findings. Labelle and Okun (1971) did not find any pathological changes in rabbit eyes light microscopically after a 6 month silicone oil filling and postulated that the other authors must have seen artifacts caused by smudging of silicone oil during cutting of the preparations. Ober et al. (1983) and Meredith et al. (1985), in further similar experiments, did not find any difference between silicone oil and control groups by light and electron microscopy either. Neither we nor any other silicone oil surgeons we know have ever seen intraretinal silicone oil inclusions, such as those reported by Jalkh and co-workers, clinically. It must be assumed that they saw emulsified silicone oil droplets in a preretinal membrane instead.

Histological investigations on enucleated eyes after silicone oil surgery, however, did show changes in the retina. In all eyes examined (Watzke 1967b, Blodi 1971, Sugar and Okamura 1976, Manschot 1978, Leaver et al. 1979b, Ni et al. 1983, Laroche et al. 1983, Parmly et al. 1986) intraretinal vacuoles were found that had probably been filled with silicone oil before preparation, during which silicone oil cannot be preserved. Cellular reactions to these suspected silicone oil inclusions were not found in any of these preparations. In one eye with massive secondary glaucoma after severe trauma coalescent globules of silicone oil were found to have infiltrated the entire length of the atrophic optic nerve, reminiscent of Schnabel's cavernous optic atrophy (Shields and Eagle 1989).

All of these eyes had, however, retinal detachments of long duration. In 1986 Kirchhof and colleagues demonstrated, on the basis of eight enucleated eyes, that such intraretinal changes only occur in detached retinas. In two of the eyes they examined, both with attached retina, and in two eyes with partial retinal detachment without subretinal silicone oil no pathological changes of the retina could be demonstrated histologically, in one of the eyes after $3^1/_2$ years of silicone oil filling. They also pointed out that the vacuoles frequently found in silicone filled eyes need not necessarily be caused by silicone oil, but may also occur in secondary spongy degeneration of the retina commonly seen in long-standing detachments.

In a further rabbit experiment Gonvers and colleagues (1986) showed that retinal changes caused by silicone oil may very well exist after all. In vitrectomized rabbit eyes they found, after a 6 week filling with silicone oil, atrophy of the outer plexiform layer in the upper parts of the retina with a clear reduction in the number of synaptic terminals. These changes could only be demonstrated in those parts of the retina that had been in permanent contact with the silicone oil bubble. At the posterior pole and in the lower retina no pathological changes were found. They performed the experiment with purified as well as normal silicone oil thinking that perhaps short molecular chains or catalytic remnants had caused these changes by a toxic chemical reaction, but the findings were identical for both silicone oils. Gonvers speculated that these changes are probably the consequence of mechanical pressure of the silicone oil bubble against the upper retina. Chang (personal communication) found an analogous effect in the lower half of the fundus during investigations with perfluorocarbons, which are heavier than water. It remains unclear though whether the human retina, the structure of which differs from that of rabbits, undergoes changes of the same kind and if so whether they would be of any clinical significance.

With the exception of Gonvers' proof of a mechanical effect of silicone oil on the upper retina, conclusive histologic evidence of a retinotoxic effect of silicone oil is still wanting.

#### 4.1.4.2 Chemistry

Refojo and colleagues (1988) found small amounts of dissolved retinol and cholesterol in a sensitive chemical analysis of silicone samples that had been removed from human eyes. They concluded that these substances probably diffused from the retina or underlying tissue into the lipophilic silicone oil. Whether this dissolution of lipids from the retina has any clinically significant effect on vision is unknown.

#### 4.1.4.3 Electrophysiology

In 1962 (a, b) Armaly produced normal electroretinograms (ERG) in owl monkeys 18 months after filling with silicone oil, but Lee and colleagues (1969) found reduced ERG responses as early as a few hours after silicone oil filling which then did not recover within a period of 2 months. This finding could not be confirmed by Ober's (1983) and Meredith's (1985) groups.

In further experimental and clinical investigations Esser et al. (1982), Momirov et al. (1983), Kirchhof et al. (1985), Foerster et al. (1985), and Thaler et al. (1986) were able to show that a reduction of both a and b waves of the ERG in eyes filled with silicone oil probably were sufficiently explained by the electrical insulating properties of silicone oil (the silicone oil General Electric SF96 used by several vitreoretinal surgeons for many years was originally developed for the filling of electric insulators on high voltage transmission lines). They all showed, furthermore, that the amplitudes of the reduced ERG potentials increased immediately after silicone oil removal in most of the eyes by more than twice the previous values and remained at just these levels thereafter. A "recovery effect" of the retina after silicone oil removal was thus improbable.

In a more recent study Kellner and colleagues (1988) examined flicker-evoked potentials as indicators of the function of the optic nerve in eyes with PVR before and after silicone oil filling. They were able to show that preoperatively missing or reduced responses to flicker stimuli increased in all eyes after silicone oil filling with retinal reattachment and did not decline again afterwards (up to 348 days). In those eyes in which the silicone oil had meanwhile been removed, these responses stayed absolutely stable as well. They concluded that the function of the optic nerve was not directly influenced by silicone oil filling. Thus, an electrophysiological indication for a possible silicone oil retinopathy is also still missing.

#### 4.1.4.4 Function of Visual Acuity

The satisfaction in the early phase of silicone oil surgery at having found a possibility of curing at least some of the retinal detachments, hopeless up to then, soon gave way to great disappointment at the often very poor visual results obtained (Watzke 1967a, Okun 1968, Cockerham et al. 1969, Kanski and Daniel 1973, Alexandridis and Daniel 1981). This experience as well as the experimental results of Lee, Mukai, Schepens, and coworkers, mentioned above, seemed to suggest that possibly silicone oil toxicity might be responsible. Functional results, however, continuously improved over the course of the years; Grey and Leaver (1979) found that the visual function in patients with attached retinas tended to remain stable. In a long-term analysis of the early cases of Okun, Chan and Okun found in 1986 that after 10 years about half of the eyes that were originally functional successes had preserved useful visual function. They concluded that early redetachment rather than late complications was usually responsible for poor visual function.

All silicone oil surgeons who published their results of vitrectomy and silicone oil in the 1980s concurred that clear clinical indications for toxicity did not exist. The analysis of our series supports these observations based on three facts:

1. *If all extraretinal factors influencing visual acuity are excluded, the average visual acuity remains stable for at least 2 years* (Figs. 17 + 18). Average visual acuity is clearly reduced by cataract after about 1 year. If only aphakic eyes are considered, the visual function, however, rises continuously for 2 years (Fig. 17). The better average visual acuity of

eyes from which the silicone oil was removed in comparison to those in which it was left in (Fig. 18) cannot be attributed to a retinotoxic effect of silicone oil either, as the difference in the curves in Fig. 18 is already present at a time when most of the eyes in both groups are still filled with oil. The final level of average visual acuity, moreover, reaches about 0.1, a level which from a clinical point of view is about what one would expect in the surgery of complicated detachments. It can thus be excluded to a large extent that visual acuities could perhaps have been improved decisively without the use of silicone oil and a possible retinotoxic effect. In our series statistical analyses beyond 2 years were not practical since there were not enough patients with attached retinas and intraocular oil left for meaningful analysis.

2. *Visual acuity with retained silicone oil may remain stable for many years.* The longest period a successfully operated on eye in our series had the oil in the eye was 6 years, and the visual acuity in that eye remained stable at 0.05 during that time in spite of a mild band keratopathy. We observed four more eyes with an attached retina and oil in the eye for more than 5 years. Three of them had a visual acuity of 0.05, the fourth reached 0.1. In the course of those 5 years we were not able to detect a tendency towards deterioration of visual acuity in any one of these four eyes either. Moreover, in the literature, there are numerous studies reporting the preservation of function for 10 (Scott 1977) and even 12 (Okun 1976) years.
3. *An analysis of the patients with loss of visual acuity despite attached retinas shows that the causes are essentially specific to the underlying disease* (Table 7). Here the most frequent causes for loss of visual acuity were atrophies of the retina and the optic nerve as would be expected for a silicone oil retinopathy. In each of these patients, however, a clear cause for the atrophy was found, and in most eyes the loss of visual acuity already occurred shortly post surgery. We could not find an explanation for bad visual performance in only 13 eyes, silicone oil retinopathy possibly being responsible in this group; nine of these 13 patients had a very short follow-up and never returned after the first discharge from the hospital so that visual acuity might meanwhile have improved. In any case long-term toxic damage by silicone oil can be excluded as an explanation in these eyes. Four eyes remain for which the poor function one is presently at a loss to explain. One patient with PVR with giant tear had a redetachment under silicone oil which was revised, and 2 months after revision visual acuity had not recovered beyond hand movement. Another eye, also with PVR and giant tear, suffered an unexplained visual deterioration from 0.05 to counting fingers 13 months after silicone oil removal. In one eye with PVR and macular hole and one with PVR and giant tear visual acuity had not recovered to more than counting fingers 3 months after successful reattachment. So

again these are not situations in which long-term toxic damage seems a likely explanation.

In summary, it can be said that after more than 20 years of experimental and clinical research no clear evidence for a retinotoxic effect of silicone oil has been found, neither histologically nor electrophysiologically nor clinically, so that at present the question of silicone oil toxicity is not discussed seriously any more. Our results show that in our patients retinal function continuously improved over a period of 2 years. In some of the eyes with retained silicone oil we found stable visual acuity for a period of 5 – 6 years.

### 4.1.5 Aphakia

There is still disagreement among silicone oil surgeons whether or not the lens should be removed in the first operation as a matter of routine even if it is clear. Lensectomy would allow better access to the vitreous base, which is necessary for the thorough dissection of anterior traction in eyes with PVR. This method was recommended by Živojnović (1987).

Due to possible complications in the anterior segment, we preserved the lens whenever possible throughout the past years and removed it only if a cataract constituted an intraoperative hindrance. When peripheral traction prevented reattachment of the retina (rare), or caused a flat peripheral, retinal redetachment postoperatively (more frequent), we relieved the traction by applying a high encircling buckle or cutting a large peripheral circumferential retinectomy.

Fig. 26 shows a comparison of the success rates in phakic and aphakic subsets of eyes. The eyes in the aphakic group either had cataract surgery preoperatively or the lens had to be removed before final silicone oil removal. Thus, at least temporarily, the oil had free access to the anterior chamber. In the phakic group the lens was either still in situ at the last follow-up examination or it was removed together with the silicone oil. Although these two groups again are statistically not quite comparable (no randomization), the curves show clearly, nevertheless, that early removal of the lens does not necessarily guarantee success. The incidence of keratopathy, however, is much lower in the phakic than in the aphakic group.

At times it may perhaps be necessary to remove a clear lens in the first operation. As a general strategy, however, the attempt to preserve the lens as long as possible offers clear advantages with regard to postoperative corneal problems and without endangering retinal reattachment to any significant degree. Ideally, we try to manage the retinal problems in phakic eyes as long as the lens is clear. We then wait for the cataract to develop and remove silicone oil and cataract at the same time. This procedure offers the additional advantage that after silicone oil removal an extracapsular cataract extraction with lens implantation in the posterior chamber remains an option.

### 4.1.6 Silicone Oil Removal

It is our aim to remove the silicone oil after successful reattachment of the retina, and in the early group this happened in 68% of the eyes. The problem is to decide when and in which eyes the oil can be removed without running undue risk of retinal redetachment.

A prerequisite for the successful removal of silicone oil is complete freedom of traction and attached retina everywhere (also peripherally). These criteria were fulfilled in all 193 silicone oil removals, but the various indication groups differed as to how quickly this point was reached. In general we removed the silicone oil earlier from eyes with either posterior holes or PDR and later from eyes with PVR or perforating injuries. The clinical know-how for selection had to be developed first, and therefore some misjudgements could not be avoided. Our redetachment rate was 14%.

Other authors also reported similar problems. Zilis et al. (1989) had a redetachment rate of 9%; Ando (1987), 15%; Federman and Schubert (1988), 16.7%; Casswell and Gregor (1987), 25%; and Cox et al. (1986), even 30%. In more than half of our retinal detachments after silicone oil removal we reattached the retina successfully. The final failure rate of 6.2% was not high enough to derive a contraindication to silicone oil removal. It reminds us, however, to continue carefully selecting those eyes from which silicone oil is to be removed, and to perform an additional revision first if traction has not been completely relieved.

As soon as the retinal situation allows and the proliferative process has remitted, after about 12 months at the latest, silicone oil removal can usually be performed. The timing, however, is influenced by a number of factors, such as cataract formation and emulsification with and without glaucoma, visual acuity, hypotony, fear of possible toxicity and of the development of proliferations in the vitreous base and on the ciliary body, and, last but not least, whether the patient is free of complaints. In practice, we performed silicone oil removal after 12.2. months on average (Fig. 20).

In some eyes the silicone oil was retained longer. Sometimes the retina was not perfectly attached or the development of cataract was not yet advanced enough. In other eyes the reason was hypotony, fear of redetachment, or logistic problems in the follow-up period which prevented renewed surgery.

The question must be asked whether silicone oil should be removed at all. Despite many years of clinical experience we find this question difficult to answer. Now as ever we aim at always removing the oil for many reasons. The long-term problems of emulsification and glaucoma probably carry the most weight. Also from a logistic point of view, we prefer to remove the silicone oil as we can only release patients without silicone oil from our regular follow-up. Further motives for removal are the aspect of toxicity, which possibly exists although we rate it low; the psychological factor that patients do not regard themselves as cured as long as oil is in the eye; and the fact that many patients can make use of their full visual potential only after silicone oil removal because of the unstable optics of the silicone oil bubble. We are, however, willing to leave the oil in for a long time provided regular follow-up is guaranteed. The problems that could arise in the long-term so far seem controllable.

Thus the following concept for silicone oil removal has crystallized: In phakic eyes we try to first treat the retinal problems, preserving the lens, and then wait for the lens to become opaque (mostly at about 12 months), removing oil and lens simultaneously. In aphakic eyes we recommend silicone oil removal at about 1 year post surgery, which we then discuss with the patient at length. After weighing the risks many patients decide to keep the oil in for a longer time and to accept the danger of an emulsification glaucoma. Since in our series considerably more eyes have been lost due to redetachment after silicone oil removal than due to long-term complications caused by the oil, such a decision is justifiable in the light of present day knowledge. We remove the oil when emulsification becomes a problem or, at the latest, when the intraocular pressure increases.

### 4.1.7 Retinectomy

It is controversial whether cutting the retina or laying large areas of the pigment epithelium free with extensive retinectomy stimulates proliferation. Increased rates of redetachment after retinectomy could be a result of the more serious pathology in those eyes, in which such retinectomies prove necessary. High failure rates might also be caused by the difficulty of tamponading large retinal defects or by the fact that retinotomy edges represent good guide structures for membrane growth. It may therefore well be possible that retinectomies have unjustly been suspected of being directly responsible for failures.

Miller and colleagues (1986a + 6b) were able to show that the wound healing behavior of the retina is determined more by intraocular inflammation and macrophage activity than by the size of the retinal wound.

In the past years we have increasingly tried to relieve anterior traction by cutting extensive circumferential retinectomies. Figure 31 shows that our success rates in eyes with PVR treated with this technique did not differ from those eyes treated without retinectomy. If retinectomies stimulated proliferation, a lower success rate would have to be expected in the retinectomy group. It is actually surprising that the failure rate in this group, which certainly includes the more complicated pathologies, was no higher than that among the more simple cases. Reproliferation after retinectomy did occur frequently but was a relatively slight clinical problem. Retinectomies that were too small initially and had to be extended in revisions procedures certainly caused more problems. Other authors have had similar experiences (Machemer et al. 1986, Haut et al. 1986, Aaberg 1988).

We have not been able to find any indication of increased proliferative activity resulting from retinal cuts. It is important though that intraocular hemorrhages are painstakingly avoided in this maneuver. since blood stimulates epiretinal membrane growth to a high degree (Miller et al. 1986c, de Juan et al. 1988). We have very occasionally experienced severe reproliferations after massive intraocular hemorrhages.

The technique of extensive retinectomies is difficult and full of risks, but it offers good chances of success. As opposed to extensive and meticulous dissection of the vitreous base, a method propagated by others for the management of severe anterior PVR (Aaberg 1988, de Juan and McCuen 1989), circumferential retinectomies allowed us to initially preserve the lens, thereby reducing the risk of complications in the anterior segment. The fear that retinectomies might cause increased proliferation is probably not justified.

## 4.2 Legal Use of Silicone Oil

To date silicone oil surgery could be looked upon as an experimental procedure for desolate cases. We have informed the patients accordingly, pointing out the experimental character of this procedure and alternative methods. All patients have preoperatively given their written consent to silicone oil filling.

From a clinical point of view, silicone oil, like other viscoelastic substances common in ophthalmologic surgery, is a surgical device and should, of course, not have any pharmacological activity if possible. The laws governing the production and prescription of pharmacological agents differ from country to country. In the USA for instance, viscoelastic substances are defined as "medical devices." According to German law and that of some other countries, however, silicone oil is defined as a pharmaceutical preparation due to its liquid nature and is therefore subject to a complete process of approval. This theoretically means that the pharmacological effect must be substantiated in clinical trials. For silicone oil such an effect probably does not and in any case should not exist. Nevertheless, using our data the German health authority (Bundesgesundheitsamt) has granted provisional permission for trial purposes and under its supervision a trial procedure is being undertaken in the form of a multicenter study, in which the clinics in Lübeck, Essen, Cologne, Würzburg, and Munich are participating. Similar trials are under way with the American FDA and in other countries. FDA approval should be imminent.

## 4.3 Alternative Substances

Despite the fact that "silicone oil", i.e., PDMS has established itself as the most useful and stable material for intraocular tamponade, the search for better alternatives has continued.

*Perfluorocarbons* with longer molecular chains (perfluoropentane, perfluoroether, perfluorotributylamine, and perfluorodecaline) are liquid substances with a surface tension and optical properties similar to silicone oil and a specific weight heavier than water (Constable 1974, Miyamoto et al. 1984+1986, Chang et al. 1987a, 1987b, 1988, 1989a+b). They are suitable therefore as an intraoperative instrument for unfolding and reattaching a detached retina without the need of a drainage retinotomy at the posterior pole (Chang et al. 1989a+b). Since their viscosity is lower than water, they emulsify massively within days; they are thus not suited for long-term tamponade and have to be removed again at the end of the operation.

*Fluorinated silicone oils* have properties very similar to PDMS (Miyamoto et al. 1986). They are, however, heavier than water and could be of advantage in PVR, since this often is more severe in the lower half of the eye, or in tamponading defects of the lower retina. First trials with polytrifluoropropylmethylsiloxane (Petersen et al. 1986, Gabel et al. 1987b, Tolentino et al. 1988) have resulted in marked inflammatory reactions so that at present these substances should not be used clinically.

Yamauchi (1984+1986) has performed preliminary experiments with a *polyvinylalcohol hydrogel* as a substitute for the vitreous body. This substance is swollen with saline, optically clear, and is well-tolerated by rabbit eyes; however, since it has by nature no surface tension towards water, its use as an intraocular tamponade is precluded in its present form.

None of the alternative substances tested so far is presently suited to replace PDMS – particularly in its purified form – as a long-term tamponade.

## 4.4 Summary

Most simple and even complicated retinal detachments can be reattached successfully with the conventional retinal and vitreous surgery methods available today. As early as the end of the 1970s it became clear, however, that in spite of modern vitreous surgical techniques some particularly complicated retinal detachments remained, in which the long-term anatomic results were disappointing. It seemed that the surgical success rates could only be improved by additional, still more aggressive surgical techniques which today are referred to as *extreme vitreoretinal surgery*. This is characterized by direct manipulation and surgery of the retina and by an intraocular long-term tamponade with long-acting gases or silicone oil.

The use of silicone oil within this extreme vitreoretinal surgery was initially to a large extent experimental, but today it is accepted in principle and is used routinely more and more in retinological centers worldwide. The Clinic for Ophthalmology in Lübeck has played an early and intensive role in the development and evaluation of silicone oil surgery and regards this subject matter as one of its centers of clinical and scientific activity. Since the development phase of silicone oil surgery has now come to a conclusion, it seemed useful to present the current state of the art and to demonstrate graphically what can be achieved by it.

The intraocularly injected silicone oil used by us (PDMS) is optically clear, lighter than water, permeable to oxygen, and has a high surface tension towards water. It is mostly chemically inert, biologically not degradable in the tissue, not carcinogenic, mechanically stable, and easily sterilizable due to its high thermal stability. Up to 1984 we used silicone oil of a viscosity of 1000 cps and, since then, a purified oil with a viscosity of 5000 cps, from which most of the short molecular chains have been removed by a special process. The German health authorities, partly on the basis of the numerical data presented in this book, have granted provisional approval for its use in clinical studies. At the same time a multicenter clinical trial in the USA is nearing completion and FDA approval seems imminent.

Due to its high surface tension silicone oil is able to tamponade retinal defects of any size safely and permanently. Thus, by its use it has become possible to perform aggressive surgical maneuvers on the retina itself, ranging from thorough delamination of epiretinal membranes to generous cutting or removal of retinal tissue under tension. In addition to tamponading retinal defects, silicone oil probably also acts as a space filler, limiting free diffusion of proliferative cells and biochemical mediators through the vitreous cavity. It mechanically inhibits the contraction of preretinal membranes, has a hemostatic effect in "tamponading" bleeding vessels, and in some cases counteracts the development of a phthisis.

Altogether 483 eyes of 463 patients having been operated on with vitrectomy and silicone oil filling between April 1981 and January 1989 in Essen and Lübeck, were entered into the analysis. Of the 483 eyes, 236 (49%) had already been operated on once or several times previously. The most frequent indication was PVR, somewhat rarer indications were giant tears, posterior holes, PDR and perforating injuries. Less frequently, eyes with nondiabetic proliferative retinopathies, acute retinal necrosis, massive subretinal hemorrhage with age-related maculopathy, and Eales' disease were operated on. In some cases indication groups overlapped. The distribution of indication groups remained essentially the same over the years, only diabetic retinopathies have clearly come to the fore and now represent about one-third of the patients coming to surgery.

The surgical procedures follow the techniques established in conventional retinal and vitreous surgery, particularly with regard to encircling band, vitrectomy, membrane peeling, and coagulation. Special maneuvers peculiar to extreme vitreoretinal surgery include peripheral circumferential retinectomies for the relief of traction, retinotomies at the posterior pole for drainage of subretinal fluid or for the removal of subretinal strands, and the use of silicone oil as an aid to fixation or for long-term tamponade. In aphakic eyes we have used an inferior basal iridectomy since 1984, through which aqueous humor can pass into the anterior chamber below the silicone oil bubble. Thus, silicone oil prolapse into the anterior chamber and secondary angle-closure and a resulting keratopathy can effectively be avoided. In the beginning silicone oil was considered a long-term tamponade not to be removed again; today it is usually removed after a few months.

Whereas in conventional retinal or vitreous surgery clinical studies are mostly concluded after 6 months, a follow-up period longer than that was aimed at because of the special problem of long-term complications caused by silicone oil. As a result of the variable length of follow-up, life table techniques were used for statistical evaluation.

In 350 of 483 eyes (72.5%) the retina was completely attached at the last follow-up examination, after 21.7 months on average. By life table analysis 76% of the operations were *anatomic successes* after 6 months. The anatomic success rate thereafter continued to fall slightly mainly due to reproliferation and stabilized at about 70% after 2 years. These results were broken down further by indication groups.

In *PVR* 103 of 144 retinas (71.5%) could be successfully reattached. This corresponded to a success rate of 75% after 6 months and 68% after 24 months by life table analysis. Most failures were due to late reproliferation.

Altogether 66% of the primarily successfully operated on eyes developed renewed retinal detachments through reproliferation, most of which, however, could be successfully revised. A review of the literature shows that the success rates in advanced stages of PVR are probably considerably better with silicone oil than with gas. Whereas silicone oil, in fact, does not prevent redetachment due to renewed proliferation, it does prevent the development of inoperable situations and often permitted us to wait with revision surgery until the proliferative process had stabilized. Our figures and observations provide no indication that silicone oil might stimulate proliferation directly.

*Giant tears* without PVR had an above average anatomic success rate of 93% absolutely and by life table analysis. Renewed retinal detachments and surgical failures could only rarely be attributed to reproliferation but rather were a result of intraoperative choroidal hemorrhage or renewed tear formation in retinal areas not involved up to then. We saw membrane formation in the sense of a PVR in 24% of the successful operations. A review of the literature shows that there is no field in retinal surgery where the success rates could be improved so dramatically in recent years as in giant tears. As compared to alternative methods, silicone oil simplifies the surgical procedure considerably and seems to prevent or at least limit the development of PVR.

With a success rate of 83% after 2 years a satisfactory result could also be achieved in *posterior holes*. Membrane formation occurred in only 11% of the eyes. Our results with macular holes show that a retinal reattachment can almost always be achieved with silicone oil and that the postoperative visual acuity is satisfactory as well. Nonetheless, since there are simpler surgical methods, silicone oil should usually not be used in the primary procedure.

After 2 years 67% of the eyes with *PDR* and traction detachment of the retina were anatomic successes by life table analysis. Renewed epiretinal membrane formation was responsible for most of the failures. It could be shown that: (a) in PDR silicone oil serves as an effective tamponade in complicated situations involving multiple or extensive retinal defects, (b) has a hemostatic effect, (c) allows quick visual rehabilitation and postoperative laser therapy where needed, (d) inhibits the development of rubeosis iridis, and (e) often prevents a painful phthisis in unsuccessfully operated eyes. Silicone oil cannot influence progressive atrophy of the retina or optic nerve despite successfully reattached retinas so that, regrettably, only about 60% of the time can we offer the patient the prospect of long-term ambulatory vision.

The clearly poorest success rates were achieved in *perforating injuries*. Whereas by life table analysis 69% of the retinas were still attached after 6 months, this value decreased to 54% after 2 years. The greatest problem with injuries of the posterior segment was the virtually unavoidable PVR which developed with particular fulminance in traumatized eyes. Silicone oil was used in eyes with perforating injuries for intraoperative or postoperative hemostasis in eyes with a high tendency to hemorrhage, as a primary filling to avoid a PVR in eyes at high risk, and in eyes with already existing PVR.

Of the 350 successfully eyes operated on, 66 (19%) did not achieve *ambulatory vision* in spite of attached retinas. Principle causes were a preexisting atrophy of the retina and the optic nerve, keratopathy, and cataract. An analysis of the *average visual acuity* in eyes with attached retinas showed a continuous improvement up to the 18th postoperative month. Although in the literature occasional hypotheses have been made as to possible toxic retinal damage by silicone oil, convincing histological, electrophysiological, or clinical indications of a retinotoxic effect of silicone oil do not exist.

An average of 2.6 operations per eye were necessary to achieve our success rates, which points to the fact that this surgical method is more suited for particularly motivated patients, i.e., primarily those with only one eye, threatened bilaterally, or after previous unsuccessful surgery.

In 193 of 362 eyes primarily successfully operated on we tried to *remove the silicone oil*. In 30 eyes (15%) problems arose postoperatively in terms of redetachment, recurrent hemorrhage, or hypotony. Of these 18 eyes could be revised successfully. The final failure rate after silicone oil removal was 6.2%. The silicone oil was generally removed between 6 and 12 months after initial surgery. The question whether silicone oil must be removed at all cannot be answered definitively despite long years of experience. In principle we aim at removing the oil from all eyes where it seems safe to do so.

Typical postoperative *complications* were cataract, emulsification, glaucoma, rubeosis iridis, and keratopathy.

Almost all phakic eyes eventually developed a *cataract*. Retaining the lens primarily for the protection of the anterior segment and removing it together with the silicone oil has proved its worth. Later we tried to implant an artificial lens in selected eyes.

Droplet formation, i.e., "*emulsification*" of the silicone oil happened in most of the eyes although with widely varying intensity. Even though our data are insufficient for statistical proof, we found clinically that the tendency to emulsification dropped considerably after introduction of the purified oil OP5000. Secondary glaucoma because of emulsification was rare and in most cases reversible after silicone oil removal.

We observed *temporary pressure increases* in 7% of the eyes successfully operated on. About half were caused by silicone oil (angle- and pupillary-block by the oil, emulsification) and, half by causes specific to the disease (chamber angle pathology, hemorrhage, inflammation). In about 11% of the successfully operated on eyes a new *persisting glau-*

*coma* developed postoperatively, usually a neovascular glaucoma in diabetic eyes. Peripheral anterior synechiae, emulsification, and protracted inflammation were also identified as probable causes. The glaucoma was well controllable medically throughout, and fistulating surgery never proved necessary. We observed a glaucomatous cupping of the optic nerve in only two eyes. Our analysis showed that secondary glaucoma after silicone oil surgery was caused by a great variety of factors. Predisposing factors, such as myopia and diabetes, secondary changes caused by the basic disease, and the surgical trauma suffered, played a far greater part than overloading of the trabecular meshwork by emulsification. Our figures demonstrate that pure "silicone oil glaucoma" is rare. Although the glaucomas were well controllable, they represent the potentially most dangerous complication with unresolved long-term problems.

We saw postoperative *rubeosis iridis* in 9% of the eyes successfully operated on. The great majority were diabetics. Due to the unfavorable initial pathology it was remarkable that this rate was so low. Our figures show that silicone oil inhibited the development of rubeosis and particularly that of neovascular glaucoma.

By life table analysis the rate of newly developed *keratopathies* was 5% after 6 months and 8% after 2 years. The incidence of keratopathy could be lowered further by the introduction of an inferior basal iridectomy in aphakic eyes. An individual analysis of the cases concerned showed that keratopathies occurred when long-term contact of silicone oil and corneal endothelium could not be prevented. This was usually due to iris defects or chronic hypotony. Even in those eyes in which a keratopathy has to be accepted, we can preserve ambulatory vision for a long time by corneal abrasion and EDTA. The fear of keratopathy is no longer a contraindication for the use of silicone oil.

A comparison of the eyes operated with and without *retinectomy* showed almost identical success rates. Considering the probably more complicated initial pathologies in those eyes in which we regarded a retinectomy as necessary, the figures demonstrate that relaxing retinectomies essentially do not influence the success rates. We were unable to find any indication of increased proliferative activity as a consequence of retinal cuts. Extensive retinectomies are technically difficult and full of risk. They offer, however, good chances of success for selected patients, and the fear of causing increased reproliferation thereby is probably not justified.

A comparison of the results of the two *main surgeons* showed essentially identical success rates. This suggests that extreme retinal surgery is a procedure that, in spite of all its complexity, can achieve reproducible results provided the equipment and the surgical techniques are the same.

With the present state of silicone oil surgery a further phase in the development of retinal detachment surgery has been completed. The methods of extreme vitreoretinal surgery using silicone oil as a long-term tamponade, which were developed primarily in Europe in recent years, enable us today to treat those retinal detachments successfully which were looked upon as inoperable only a few years ago. The principles and procedures have been standardized to quite an extent and can be improved further only in detail. Future possibilities for further improvements will probably be found in prevention and in supplementary pharmacological therapy. In many diabetics advanced stages of PDR could, for instance, be effectively prevented by adequate and timely laser treatment, and the incidence of PVR could be reduced by improved primary care of uncomplicated retinal detachments. Pharmacological agents for the prevention or inhibition of proliferative membrane growth are still in the developmental stages, and it cannot be foreseen whether and when they will be clinically applicable. The future will show to what extent further progress can actually be made.

# References

1. Aaberg TM, Blair CJ, Gass JDM: Macular holes. Am J Ophthalmol, 69 (1970) 555-562

2. Aaberg TM: Clinical results in vitrectomy for diabetic traction retinal detachment. Am J Ophthalmol, 88 (1979) 246-253

3. Aaberg TM: Management of anterior and posterior proliferative vitreoretinopathy. XLV Edward Jackson Memorial Lecture Am J Ophthalmol, 106 (1988) 519-532

4. Aaberg TM: Postoperative response after diabetic vitrectomy; clinical characteristics, anatomical and functional results, risk factors and new treatment modalities. 6thVail vitreoretinal seminar, Vail, (1989) March 12 – 19

5. Abrams GW, Topping TM, Machemer R: Vitrectomy for injury. The effect on intraocular proliferation following perforation of the posterior segment of the rabbit eye. Arch Ophthalmol, 97 (1979) 743-748

6. Abrams GW, Swanson DE, Sabates WI, Goldman AI: The results of sulfur hexafluoride gas in vitreous surgery. Am J Ophthalmol, 94 (1982) 165-171

7. Abrams GW, Williams GA, Neuwirth J, McDonald HR: Clinical results of titanium retinal tacks with pneumatic insertion. Am J Ophthalmol, 102 (1986) 13-19

8. Alexandridis E, Daniel H: Results of silicone oil injection into the vitreous. Dev Ophthalmol, 2 (1981) 24-27

9. Anand R, Fisher DH: Silicone oil in the management of retinal detachment with acute retinal necrosis. In: Proliferative vitreoretinopathie (PVR). Springer, Berlin Heidelberg New York (1988) 169-176

10. Ando F, Kondo J: A plastic tack for the treatment of retinal detachment with giant tear. Am J Ophthalmol, 95 (1983) 260

11. Ando F: Usefulness and limit of silicone oil in the management of complicated retinal detachment. Jpn J Ophthalmol, 31 (1987) 138-146

12. Ando F, Miyakawa N, Nagasaka T, Sekiryu T, Nonomura K, Masago A: Postoperative visual function of retinal detachment with macular hole treated with a simplified buckling procedure. 16th Meeting of the Club Jules Gonin, Bruge (1988) Sept, 4 – 9

13. Antoszyk AN, McCuen BW II, de Juan E, Machemer R Silicone oil injection after failed primary vitreous surgery in severe ocular trauma. Am J Ophthalmol, 107 (1989) 537-543

14. Armaly MF: Ocular tolerance to silicones. Arch Ophthalmol, 68 (1962) 390-395

15. Armaly MF: More ocular uses of silicone forms. Invest Ophthalmol Vis Sci, 1 (1962) 434

16. Barry PJ, Hiscott PS, Grierson I, Marshall J, McLeod D: Reparative epiretinal fibrosis after diabetic vitrectomy. Trans Ophthalmol Soc UK, 104 (1985) 287-298

17. Beekhuis WH, van Rij G, Živojnović R: Silicone oil keratopathy: indications for keratoplasty. Br J Ophthalmol, 69 (1985) 247-253

18. Benson, Machemer R: Severe perforating injuries treated with pars plana vitrectomy. Am J Ophthalmol, 81 (1976) 728-732

19. Billington BM, Leaver PK: Vitrectomy and fluid/silicone oil exchange for giant retinal tears: results at 18 months. Graefe's Arch Clin Exp Ophthalmol, 224 (1986) 7-10

20. Binder S, Velikay M, Zügner M, Stolba U, Wedrich A: Zum Sekundärglaukom nach Silikonölimplantation: Indikation, Technik und Ergebnisse. Spektrum Augenheilkd, 2/5 (1988) 224-227

21. Binder S, Velikay M, Stolba U, Kulnig W: High energy electron radiation used to inhibit intraocular proliferation: an experimental and clinical study. International symposium on PVR, Cologne (1988) Sept 1– 2

22. Birch-Hirschfeld A cited in Liesenhoff 1968 Arch Ophthalmol, 82 (1912) 241-299

23. Blankenship GW: Endophthalmitis after vitrectomy. Am J Ophthalmol, 84 (1977) 815-817

24. Blankenship GW, Machemer R: Pars plana vitrectomy for the management of severe diabetic retinopathy: An analysis of results five years following surgery. Trans Am Acad Ophthalmol Otolaryngol, 85 (1978) 553-559

25. Blankenship GW, Ibanez-Langlois S: Treatment of myopic macular hole and detachment. Ophthalmology, 94 (1987) 333-336

26. Blodi FC: Injection and impregnation of liquid silicone into ocular tissues. Am J Ophthalmol, 71 (1971) 1044-1051

27. Blumenkranz MS, Hernandez E, Ophir A, Norton EWD: 5-Fluorouracil. New applications in complicated retinal detachment for an established antimetabolite. Ophthalmology, 91 (1984) 122-130

28. Blumenkranz MS, Culbertson WW, Clarkson JG, Dix R: Treatment of the acute retinal necrosis syndrome with intravenous acyclovir. Ophthalmology, 93 (1986) 296-300

29. Blumenkranz MS, Clarkson J, Culbertson WW, Flynn HW, Lewis ML, Young AM: Vitrectomy for retinal detachment associated with acute retinal necrosis. Am J Ophthalmol, 106 (1988) 426-429

30. Bonnet I: Essais de traitement de certains décollements de rétine par injection de silicone intra-vitréen. Bull Soc Ophtalmol France, 64 (1964) 451-453

31. Bornfeld N, El-Hifnawi E, Laqua H: Ultrastructural characteristics of preretinal membranes from human eyes filled with liquid silicone. Am J Ophthalmol, 103 (1987) 770-775

32. Brinton GS, Aaberg TM, Reeser FH, Topping TM, Abrams GW: Surgical results in ocular trauma involving the posterior segment. Am J Ophthalmol, 93 (1982) 271-278

33. Brodrick JD: Keratopathy following retinal detachment surgery. Arch Ophthalmol, 96 (1978) 2021-2026

34. Brourman ND, Blumenkranz MS, Cox MS, Trese MT: Silicone oil for the treatment of severe proliferative diabetic retinopathy. Ophthalmology, 96 (1989) 759-764

35. Burke JM, McDonald R, Neuwirth J, Lewandowski M: Titanium retinal tacks with pneumatic insertion. Histologic evaluation in rabbits. Arch Ophthalmol, 105 (1987) 404-408

36. Campochiaro PA, Kaden IH, Vidaurri-Leal J, Glaser BM: Cryotherapy enhances intravitreal dispersion of viable retinal pigment epithelial cells. Arch Ophthalmol, 103 (1985) 434-436

37. Casswell AG, Gregor ZJ: Silicone oil removal. II. Operative and postoperative complications. Br J Ophthalmol, 71 (1987) 898-902

38. Champion R, Faulborn J, Bowald S, Erb P: Peritoneal reaction to liquid silicone: an experimental study. Graefe's Arch Clin Exp Ophthalmol, 225 (1987) 141-145

39. Chan C-C, Okun E: The question of ocular tolerance to intravitreal liquid silicone. Ophthalmology, 93 (1986) 651-660

40. Chandler DB, H ida T, Sheta S, Proia AD, Machemer R Improvement in efficacy of corticosteroid therapy in an animal model of proliferative vitreoretinopathy by pretreatment. Graefe's Arch Clin Exp Ophthalmol, 225 (1987) 259-265

41. Chang S, Coleman DJ, Lincoff H, Wilcox LM, Braunstein RA, Maisel JM: Perfluoropropane gas in the management of proliferative vitreoretinopathy. Am J Ophthalmol, 98 (1984) 180-188

42. Chang S, Lincoff H, Coleman J, Fuchs W, Matthew E, Jackson D: Perfluorocarbon gases in vitreous surgery. Ophthalmology, 92 (1985) 651-656

43. Chang S, Zimmermann NJ, Iwamoto T, Ortiz R, Faris D: Experimental vitreous replacement with perfluorobutylamine. Am J Ophthalmol, 103 (1987) 29-37

44. Chang S: Low viscosity liquid fluorochemicals in vitreous surgery. Am J Ophthalmol, 103 (1987) 38-43

45. Chang S: Intraoperative perfluorocarbon liquids in the management of proliferative vitreoretinopathy. Am J Ophthalmol, 106 (1988) 668-674

46. Chang S, Lincoff H, Zimmerman NJ, Fuchs W: Giant retinal tears. Surgical techniques and results using perfluorocarbon liquids. Arch Ophthalmol, 107 (1989) 761-766

47. Chang S, Repucci V, Zimmerman NJ, Heinemann M-H, Coleman J: Perfluorocarbon liquids in the management of traumatic retinal detachments. Ophthalmology, 96 (1989) 785-792

48. Charles S: Vitrectomy for retinal detachment. Trans Ophthalmol Soc UK, 10 (1980) 542-549

49. Charles S: Vitreous microsurgery. Williams and Wilkins, Baltimore, (1981)

50. Chen JC: Pars plana reconstructive surgery in penetrating injury. Ann Ophthalmol, 15 (1983) 1034-1044

51. Chignell AH, Clement RS, Revie IHS: Pigment fallout and uveitis after cryotherapy. Br J Ophthalmol, 57 (1973) 156-165

52. Chong LP, de Juan E, McCuen BW II, Landers MB III: Endophthalmitis in a silicone oil-filled eye. Am J Ophthalmol, 102 (1986) 660

53. Chung H, Tolentino FI, Cajita VN, Acosta J, Refojo MF: Reevaluation of corneal complications after closed vitrectomy. Arch Ophthalmol, 106 (1988) 916-919

54. Cibis PA, Becker B, Okun E, Canaan S: The use of liquid silicone in retinal detachment. Arch Ophthalmol, 68 (1962) 590-599

55. Cibis PA: Vitreous transfer and silicone injections. Trans Am Acad Ophthalmol Otolaryngol, 68 (1964) 983-987

56. Cibis PA: Recent methods in the surgical treatment of retinal detachment. Trans Ophthalmol Soc UK, 85 (1965) 111-127

57. Cibis PA: Vitreoretinal pathology and surgery in retinal detachment. Mosby, St. Louis (1965)

58. Cinotti AA, Maltzmon BA: Prognosis and treatment of perforating ocular injuries. Ophthalmic Surg, 6 (1975) 54-61

59. Cleary PE, Ryan SJ: Method of production and natural history of experimental posterior penetrating eye injury in the rhesus monkey. Am J Ophthalmol, 88 (1979) 212-220

60. Clemens, Kroll P, Busse H, Berg P: Ultrasonography as a routine examination before treatment of retinal detachment due to macular hole. Graefe's Arch Clin Exp Ophthalmol, 224 (1986) 226-229

61. Cockerham WD, Schepens CL, Freeman HM: Silicone injection in retinal detachment. Mod Probl Ophthal, 8 (1969) 525-540

62. Coleman DJ: Early vitrectomy in the management of the severely traumatized eye. Am J Ophthalmol, 93 (1982) 543-551

63. Coleman DJ, Lucas BC, Fleischman JA, Dennis PH, Chang S, Iwamoto T, Nalbandian RM: A biological tissue adhesive for vitreoretinal surgery. Retina, 8 (1988) 250-256

64. Constable IJ: Perfluoropentane in experimental ocular surgery. Invest Ophthalmol Vis Sci, 13 (1974) 627-629

65. Cox MS, Trese MT, Murphy PL: Silicone oil for advanced proliferative vitreoretinopathy. Ophthalmology, 93 (1986) 646-650

66. Crisp A, de Juan E, Tiedemann J: Effect of silicone oil viscosity on emulsification. Arch Ophthalmol, 105 (1987) 546-550

67. Custodis E: Bedeutet die Plombenaufnähung auf die Sklera einen Fortschritt in der operativen Behandlung der Netzhautablösung? Ber Dtsch Ophthalmol Ges, 58 (1953) 102-110

68. Cutler NL: Transplantation of human vitreous. Arch Ophthalmol, 35 (1946) 615-623

69. Cutler SJ, Ederer F: Maximum utilization of the life table method in analyzing survival. J Chronic Dis, 8 (1958) 699-712

70. de Bustros S, Glaser BM, Jonson MA: Thrombin infusion for the control of intraocular bleeding during vitreous surgery. Arch Ophthalmol, 103 (1985) 837-839

71. de Bustros S, Thompson JT, Michels R.G, Rice TA, Glaser BM: Vitrectomy for idiopathic epiretinal membranes causing macular pucker. Br J Ophthalmol, 72 (1988) 692-695

72. de Corral LR, Peyman GA: Pars plana vitrectomy and intravitreal silicone oil injection in eyes with rubeosis iridis. Can J Ophthalmol, 21 (1986) 10-12

73. de Juan E, Hickingbotham D, Machemer E: Retinal tacks. Am J Ophthalmol, 99 (1985) 272-274

74. de Juan E, McCuen BW II, Machemer R: The use of retinal tacks in the repair of complicated retinal detachments. Am J Ophthalmol, 102 (1986) 20-24

75. de Juan E, Hardy M, Hatchell D, Hatchell M: The effect of intraocular silicone oil on anterior chamber oxygen pressure in cats. Arch Ophthalmol, 104 (1986) 1063-1064

76. de Juan E, Dickson JS, Hjelmeland L: Serum is chemotactic for retinal-derived glial cells. Arch Ophthalmol, 106 (1988) 986-990

77. de Juan E, McCuen BW II: Management of anterior vitreous traction in proliferative vitreoretinopathy. Retina, 9 (1989) 258-262

78. Dellaporta A: Endodiathermy for retinal detachment with macular hole. Am J Ophthalmol, 95 (1983) 405-407

79. Deutmann AF, Eijkenboom GJM, Fanuriakis C: A microsurgical method for the injection of intraocular silicone oil. Int Ophthalmol, 2 (1980) 63-69

80. Deutschmann R: Zur operativen Behandlung der Netzhautablösung. Klin Monats Augenheilkd, 1 (1906) 364-370

81. Diddie KR, Stern WH, Ober RR, et al: Intraocular silicone oil for recurrent proliferative vitreoretinopathy in vitrectomized eyes. ARVO Abstracts Invest Ophthalmol Vis Sci, 24(Suppl) (1983) 173

82. Dimopoulos S, Heimann K: Spätkomplikationen nach Silikonölinjektion. Langzeitbeobachtungen an 100 Fällen. Klin Monats Augenheilkd, 189 (1986) 223-227

83. Durlu YK, Ishiguro S, Yoshida A, Mito T, Tsuchiya M, Tamai M: Response of Müller cells following experimental lensectomy-vitrectomy. Graefe's Arch Clin Exp Ophthalmol, 228 ()1990 44-48

84. Eckardt C, Hennig G: Transsklerale Magnet-Fixierung der Netzhaut bei komplizierter Amotio. Klin Monats Augenheilkd, 185 (1984) 296-298

85. Eckardt C: Tierexperimentelle Untersuchungen zur Linsentrübung bei temporärer intraokularer Silikonauffüllung. 84. Tagung der Deutschen Ophthalmologischen Gesellschaft, Aachen (1986) Sept 21 – 24

86. Ederer F: Shall we count numbers of eyes or number of subjects? Arch Ophthalmol, 89 (1973) 1-2

87. Emmerich K-H, Meyer-Rüsenberg H-W, Busse H Fibrin-retinopexy. International symposium on PVR, Cologne (1988) Sept 1– 2

88. Esser J, Foerster MH, Laqua H: ERG-Befunde bei Patienten mit intraokularer Silikonöl-Füllung. Fortschr Ophthalmol, 80 (1982) 128-129

89. Failer J, Faulborn J, Erb P: Die Phagozytose von Silikonölen unterschiedlicher Viskosität durch Peritoneal-Makrophagen der Maus. Klin Monats Augenheilkd, 184 (1984) 450-452

90. Fastenberg DM, Diddie KR, Delmage JM, Dorey K: Intraocular injection of silicone oil for experimental proliferative vitreoretinopathy. Am J Ophthalmol, 95 (1983) 663-667

91. Faulborn J, Olivier D, Atkinson A: Präventive Chirurgie bei der Versorgung schwerverletzter Augen; Spätergebnisse, Komplikationen, Nachbehandlung. Klin Monats Augenheilkd, 169 (1976) 562-569

92. Faulborn J, Topping TM: Proliferations in the vitreous cavity after perforating injuries. A histopathological study. Graefe's Arch Clin Exp Ophthalmol, 205 (1978) 157-166

93. Faulborn J: Indikation zur Silikonölimplantation bei fortgeschrittener proliferativer diabetischer Retinopathie. Klin Monats Augenheilkd, 185 (1984) 362-363

94. Faulborn J, Bowald S: The vitreous after C3F8 gas instillation: long term histologic findings after spontaneous reabsorption of the gas in the rabbit. Graefe's Arch Clin Exp Ophthalmol, 225 (1987) 99-102

95. Federman JL, Shakin JL, Lanning RC: The microsurgical management of giant retinal tears with transcleral retinal sutures. Ophthalmology, 89 (1982) 832-839

96. Federman JL, Schubert HD: Complications associated with the use of silicone oil in 150 eyes after retina-vitreous surgery. Ophthalmology, 95 (1988) 870-876

97. Fineberg E, Machemer R, Sullivan P, Norton EWD, Hamasaki D, Anderson D: Sulfur hexafluoride in owl monkey vitreous cavity. Am J Ophthalmol, 79 (1975) 67-74

98. Fisher YL, Shakin JL, Slakter JS, Sorenson JA, Shafer DM: Perfluoropropane gas, modified panretinal photocoagulation and vitrectomy in the management of severe proliferative vitreoretinopathy. Arch Ophthalmol, 106 (1988) 1255-1260

99. Flynn HW, Lee WG, Parel J-M: A simple extrusion needle with flexible cannula tip for vitreoretinal microsurgery. Am J Ophthalmol, 105 (1988) 215-216

100. Foerster MH, Esser J, Laqua H: Silicone oil and its influence on electrophysiologic findings. Am J Ophthalmol, 99 (1985) 201-206

101. Foerster MH, Bornfeld N, Messmer E, Wessing A Silicone oil and secondary reproliferation in proliferative vitreoretinopathy. International symposium on PVR, Cologne (1988) Sept 1– 2

102. Foos RY: Nonvascular proliferative extraretinal retinopathies. Am J Ophthalmol, 86 (1978) 723-725

103. Foulks GN, de Juan E, Hatchell DL, McAdoo T, Hardin J: The effect of perfluoropropane on the cornea in rabbits and cats. Arch Ophthalmol, 105 (1987) 256-259

104. Freeman HM, Castillejos ME: Current management of giant retinal breaks: results with vitrectomy and total air fluid exchange in 95 cases. Trans Am Ophthalmol Soc, 79 (1981) 89-100

105. Friberg TR: The effect of vitreous and retinal surgery on corneal endothelial cell density. Ophthalmology, 91 (1984) 1166-1169

106. Fritz MH: The substitution of cerebrospinal fluid for vitreous clouded with opacities. Am J Ophthalmol, 30 (1947) 979-984

107. Fung WE, Hall DL, Cleasby GW: Combined technique for a 355 degree traumatic giant retinal break. Arch Ophthalmol, 93 (1975) 264-266

108. Gabel V-P, Kampik A, Burkhardt J: Analysis of intraocularly applied silicone oils of various origins. Graefe's Arch Clin Exp Ophthalmol, 225 (1987) 160-162

109. Gabel V-P, Kampik A, Gabel C,, Spiegel D: Silicone oil with high specific gravity for intraocular use. Br J Ophthalmol, 71 (1987) 262-267

110. Galezowski X: Du décollement de la rétine et de son traitement. Recueil Ophthalmol, 12 (1890) 1-3

111. Gao R, Neubauer L, Tang S, Kampik A Silicone oil in the anterior chamber. Graefe's Arch Clin Exp Ophthalmol, 227 (1989) 106-109

112. Gnad HD, Skorpik C, Paroussis P, Radda TM, Klemen UM, Lessel MR, Thaler A: Funktionelle und anatomische Resultate nach temporärer Silikonimplantation. Klin Monats Augenheilkd, 185 (1984) 364-367

113. Gnad HD, Skorpik C, Paroussis P,Menapace R,Radda TM,Prskavec FH,Grasl M: Temporäre Silikonöl-Implantation nach Vitrektomie bei proliferativer diabetischer Retinopathie. Klin Monats Augenheilkd, 189 (1986) 388-390

114. Gonin J: Guérisons opératoires des décollements retiniens. Rev Gen Ophthalmol, 37 (1923) 295-322

115. Gonvers M: Temporary use of intraocular silicone oil in the treatment of detachment with massive periretinal proliferation. Ophthalmologica, 184 (1982) 210-218

116. Gonvers M, Machemer R: A new approach to treating retinal detachment with macular hole. Am J Ophthalmol, 94 (1982) 468-472

117. Gonvers M: Temporary use of silicone oil in the treatment of proliferative vitreoretinopathy. Graefe's Arch Clin Exp Ophthalmol, 221 (1983) 46-53

118. Gonvers M: Temporary silicone oil tamponade in the management of retinal detachment with proliferative vitreoretinopathy. Am J Ophthalmol, 100 (1985) 239-245

119. Gonvers M, Hornung JP, de Courten C: The effect of liquid silicone on the rabbit retina. Histologic and ultrastructural study. Arch Ophthalmol, 104 (1986) 1057-1062

120. Grey RHB, Leaver PK: Results of silicone oil injection in massive preretinal retraction. Trans Ophthalmol Soc UK, 97 (1977) 238-241

121. Grey RHB, Leaver PK: Silicone oil in the treatment of massive preretinal retraction. I. Results in 105 eyes. Br J Ophthalmol, 63 (1979) 355-360

122. Grizzard WS, Hilton GF: Scleral buckling for retinal detachment complicated by periretinal proliferation. Arch Ophthalmol, 100 (1982) 419-422

123. Grossman K cited in Liesenhoff 1968 OphthRev, (1883) 288

124. Grossniklaus HE, Wood WJ, Bargeron CB, Green WR: Sulfur and calcific keratopathy associated with retinal detachment surgery and vitrectomy. Ophthalmology, 93 (1986) 260-264

125. Habal MB, Powell ML, Schimpff RD: Immunological evaluation of the tumorigenic response to implanted polymers. J Biomed Mater Res, 14 (1980) 455-466

126. Haimann MH, Burton TC, Brown CK: Epidemiology of retinal detachment. Arch Ophthalmol, 100 (1982) 289-292

127. Han DP, Mieler WF, Abrams GW, Williams GA: Vitrectomy for traumatic retinal incarceration. Arch Ophthalmol, 106 (1988) 640-645

128. Haut J, Ullern M, Chermet M, van Effenterre G: Complications of intraocular injections of silicone combined with vitrectomy. Ophthalmologica, 180 (1980) 29-35

129. Haut J, Ullern M, Chermet M, van Effenterre G: Complications des injections intra-oculaires de silicone. Bull Soc Ophtalmol Fr, 80 (1980) 519-523

130. Haut J, Larricart P, Geant G, van Effenterre G, Vachet JM: Circular subtotal retinectomy and inferior semicircular retinotomy. Ophthalmologica, 192 (1986) 129-134

131. Hayano S, Voschino S: Lokale Anwendung von Polyvinylpyrrolidon bei einigen Augenerkrankungen. J Clin Ophthalmol Jap, 13 (1959) 449-453

132. Heimann K, Paulmann H, Tavakolian U: Indikationen zur Pars-plana-Vitrektomie bei perforierenden Augenverletzungen. Klin Monats Augenheilkd, 172 (1978) 263-269

133. Heimann K, Tavakolian U, Paulmann H: Die Bedeutung der Pars-plana-Vitrektomie in der Behandlung von Verletzungen im hinteren Augenabschnitt. Sitzungsbericht der 136. Versammlung der Rhein-Westfälischen Augenärzte, (1979) 35-42

134. Heimann K: Zur Behandlung komplizierter Riesenrisse der Netzhaut. Klin Monats Augenheilkd, 176 (1980) 491-492

135. Heimann K, Dimopolous S: Intra- und postoperative Komplikationen bei Silikonölinjektion zur Behandlung komplizierter Netzhautablösungen. Klin Monats Augenheilkd, 185 (1984) 371-372

136. Heimann K, Dimopoulos S, Paulmann H: Silikonölinjektion in der Behandlung komplizierter Netzhautablösungen. Klin Monats Augenheilkd, 185 (1984) 505-508

137. Heimann K, Dahl B, Dimopoulos S, Lemmen KD: Pars plana vitrectomy and silicone oil injection in proliferative diabetic retinopathy. Graefe's Arch Clin Exp Ophthalmol, 227 (1989) 152-156

138. Hilton G, Grizzard WS: Pneumatic retinopexy. A two-step outpatient operation without conjunctival incision. Ophthalmology, 93 (1986) 626-641

139. Ho PC, McMeel JW: Retinal detachment with proliferative vitreoretinopathy: surgical results with scleral buckling, closed vitrectomy, and intravitreous air injection. Br J Ophthalmol, 69 (1985) 584-587

140. Howard RO, Campbell CJ: Surgical repair of retinal detachments caused by macular holes. Arch Ophthalmol, 81 (1969) 317-321

141. Howard RO, Gaasterland DE: Giant retinal dialysis and tear. Arch Ophthalmol, 84 (1970) 312-315

142. Höpping W: Lichtkoagulation nach Glaskörperersatz durch Silikon. Ber Dtsch Ophthalmol Ges, 66 (1964) 336-342

143. Hruby K: Hyaluronsäure als Glaskörperersatz bei Netzhautablösung. Klin Monats Augenheilkd, 138 (1961) 484-496

144. Hutton WL, Fuller DG: Factors influencing final visual results in severely injured eyes. Am J Ophthalmol, 97 (1984) 715-722

145. Hutton WL: Intraocular gases in the management of proliferative vitreoretinopathy. International symposium on PVR, Cologne (1988) Sept 1–2

146. Jaffe MJ, Oliver MS, von Fricken MA, Silberstein L, Wyatt RJ: A screening method using tissue culture for evaluation of potential retinal adhesives. Retina, 9 (1989) 328-333

147. Jalkh AE, Avila MP, Schepens CL, Azzolini C, Duncan JE, Trempe CL: Surgical treatments of proliferative vitreoretinopathy. Arch Ophthalmol, 102 (1984) 1135-1139

148. Jalkh AE, McMeel JW, Kozlowski IMD, Schepens CL: Silicone oil retinopathy. Arch Ophthalmol, 104 (1986) 178-179

149. Johnson RN, Flynn HW, Parel J-M, Portugal LM Transient hypopion with marked anterior chamber fibrin following pars plana vitrectomy and silicone oil injection. Arch Ophthalmol, 107 (1989) 683-686

150. Kanski JJ, Daniel R: Intravitreal silicone injection in retinal detachment. Br J Ophthalmol, 57 (1973) 542-545

151. Kanski JJ: Giant retinal tears. Am J Ophthalmol, 79 (1975) 847-852

152. Karel I, Filipec M, Obenberger J: Specular microscopy of the corneal endothelium after liquid silicone injection into the vitreous in complicated retinal detachments. Graefe's Arch Clin Exp Ophthalmol, 224 (1986) 195-200

153. Kasner D, Miller Gr, Taylor WH, Sever RJ, Norton EWD: Surgical treatment of amyloidosis of the vitreous. Trans Am Acad Ophthalmol Otolaryngol, 72 (1968) 410-416

154. Kellner U, Lucke K, Foerster MH: Effect of intravitreal liquid silicone on optic nerve function. Am J Ophthalmol, 106 (1988) 293-297

155. Kirchhof B, Tavakolian U, Heimann K: Histopathological and electrophysiological findings in eyes after silicone oil injection. Int Ophthalmol, 8 (1985) 94-99

156. Kirchhof B, Tavakolian U, Paulmann H, Heimann K: Histopathological findings in eyes after silicone oil injection. Graefe's Arch Clin Exp Ophthalmol, 224 (1986) 34-37

157. Kirkby GR, Gregor ZJ: The removal of silicone oil from the anterior chamber in phakic eyes. Arch Ophthalmol, 105 (1987) 1592

158. Kirmani M, Santana M, Sorgente N, Wiedemann P, Ryan SJ: Anti-proliferative drugs in the treatment of experimental proliferative vitreoretinopathy. Control by daunomycin. Retina, 3 (1983) 269-275

159. Klemen UM, Freyler H, Gnad HD, Prskavec FH: Risikofaktoren für die Entstehung einer Rubeosis iridis nach Vitrektomien beim Diabetiker. Klin Monats Augenheilkd, 179 (1981) 505-507

160. Klöti R: Vitrektomie I. Ein neues Instrument für die hintere Vitrektomie. Albrecht von Graefe's Arch Ophthalmol, 187 (1973) 161-166

161. Klöti R: Silver clip for central retinal detachment with macular hole. Mod Probl Ophthal, 12 (1974) 330-336

162. Körner F, Merz A, Gloor B, Wagner E Postoperative retinal fibrosis – a controlled clinical study of systemic steroid therapy. Graefe's Arch Clin Exp Ophthalmol, 219 (1982) 268-271

163. Krampitz-Glaas G, Laqua H Pars-plana-Vitrektomie bei der proliferativen diabetischen Retinopathie. Klin Monats Augenheilkd, 188 (1986) 283-287

164. Kreiner CF: Chemical and physical aspects of clinically applied silicones. Dev Ophthal, 14 (1987) 11-19

165. Kroll P, Busse H, Berg P, Clemens S: Intraokulare Therapie makulalochbedingter Netzhautveränderungen. Klin Monats Augenheilkd, 187 (1985) 499-502

166. Kroll P, Meyer-Rüsenberg HW, Busse H: Vorschlag zur Stadieneinteilung der proliferativen diabetischen Retinopathie. Fortschr Ophthalmol, 84 (1987) 360-363

167. Kroll P, Berg P, Biermeyer H: Langzeitergebnisse nach vitreoretinaler Silikonölchirurgie. Fortschr Ophthalmol, 85 (1988) 259-262

168. Kroll P, Gerding H, Biermeyer H Time course of reproliferations after vitrectomy and silicone oil injection in relation to primary retinal disease. International symposium on PVR, Cologne (1988) Sept 1– 2

169. Labelle P, Okun E: Ocular tolerance to liquid silicone. An experimental study. Can J Ophthalmol, 7 (1971) 199-204

170. Lambrou FH, Burke JM, Aaberg TM: Effect of silicone oil on experimental traction retinal detachment. Arch Ophthalmol, 105 (1987) 1269-1272

171. Laqua H, Machemer R: Clinical pathological correlation in massive periretinal proliferation. Am J Ophthalmol, 80 (1975) 913-929

172. Laqua H: Intravitreale Gastamponade zur Behandlung ausgewählter Netzhautablösungen. Klin Monats Augenheilkd, 175 (1979) 32-39

173. Laqua H: Collagen formation by periretinal cellular membranes. Dev Ophthal, 2 (1981) 396-406

174. Laqua H, Herwig M, Wessing A, Meyer-Schwickerath G: Silikon-Öl-Injektion zur Behandlung komplizierter Netzhautablösungen. Fortschr Ophthalmol, 79 (1982) 233-235

175. Laqua H, Wessing A: Riesenrisse der Netzhaut. Fortschr Ophthalmol, 80 (1983) 322-323

176. Laqua H: Die Behandlung der Ablatio mit Makulaforamen nach der Methode von Gonvers und Machemer. Klin Monats Augenheilkd, 186 (1985) 13-17

177. Laqua H, Lucke K, Foerster MH: Results of silicone oil surgery. Jpn J Ophthalmol, 31 (1987) 124-131

178. Laroche L, Pavlakis C, Saraux H, Orcel L: Ocular findings following intravitreal silicone injection. Arch Ophthalmol, 101 (1983) 1422-1425

179. Lean JS, Leaver PK, Cooling RG, McLeod D: The management of complex retinal detachment by pars plana vitrectomy and silicone oil. Trans Ophthalmol Soc UK, 2 (1982) 203-205

180. Lean JS, Van Der Zee WAM, Ryan SJ: Experimental model of proliferative vitreoretinopathy in the vitrectomised eye: effect of silicone oil. Br J Ophthalmol, 68 (1984) 332-335

181. Leaver PK, Cleary PE: Macular hole and retinal detachment. Trans Ophthalmol Soc UK, 95 (1975) 145-147

182. Leaver PK, Grey RHB, Garner A: Complications following silicone oil injection. Mod Probl Ophthal, 20 (1979) 290-294

183. Leaver PK, Grey RHB, Garner A: Silicone oil injection in the treatment of massive preretinal retraction. II. Late complications in 93 eyes. Br J Ophthalmol, 63 (1979) 361-367

184. Lee PF, Donovan RH, Mukai N, Schepens C, McKenzie-Freeman HM: Intravitreous injection of silicone. An experimental study. I. Clinical picture and histology of the eye. Ann Ophthalmol, 1 (1969) 15-25

185. Lemmen KD, Michel K, Kirchhof B, Paulmann H, Heimann K: Klinische und morphologische Aspekte der Silikon-Keratopathie im Tierexperiment. Fortschr Ophthalmol, 82 (1985) 556-558

186. Lemmen KD, Dimopoulos S, Kirchhof B, Heimann K: Keratopathy following pars plana vitrectomy with silicone oil filling. Dev Ophthal, 13 (1987) 88-98

187. Lemmen KD, Heimann K: Früh-Vitrektomie mit primärer Silikonölinjektion bei schwerstverletzten Augen. Klin Monats Augenheilkd, 193 (1988) 594-601

188. Lemmen KD, Kosch G, Heidner K, Heimann K: Influence of vitreous substitute on the results of early vitrectomy in experimental severe posterior segment trauma. 16th Meeting of the Club Jules Gonin, Bruge (1988) Sept, 4 – 9

189. Lemor M, Yeo JH, Glaser BM: Oral colchicine for the treatment of experimental traction retinal detachment. Arch Ophthalmol, 104 (1987) 1226-1229

190. Levine AM, Ellis RA: Intraocular liquid silicone implants. Am J Ophthalmol, 55 (1963) 939-943

191. Lewis H, Aaberg TA, Packo KH, Richmond PP, Blumenkranz MS, Blankenship GW: Intrusion of retinal tacks. Am J Ophthalmol, 103 (1987) 672-680

192. Lewis H, Aaberg TM: Anterior proliferative vitreoretinopathy. Am J Ophthalmol, 105 (1988) 277-284

193. Lewis H, Burke JM, Abrams GW, Aaberg TM: Perisilicone proliferation after vitrectomy for proliferative vitreoretinoathy. Ophthalmology, 95 (1988) 583-591

194. Liesenhoff H: Über eine verbesserte Technik bei der Silikoninjektion in den Glaskörperraum während der Ablatio-Operation. Klin Monats Augenheilkd, 152 (1968) 658-665

195. Lincoff A, Lincoff H, IwamotoT, Jacobiec F, Kreissing I: Perfluoro-n-butane. A gas for a maximum duration retinal tamponade. Arch Ophthalmol, 101 (1983) 460-462

196. Lincoff H, McLean JM, Nano H: Cryosurgical treatment of retinal detachment. Trans Am Acad Ophthalmol Otolaryngol, 68 (1964) 412-416

197. Lincoff H, Baras I, McLean J: Modifications to the Custodis procedure for retinal detachment. Arch Ophthalmol, 73 (1965) 160-166

198. Lincoff H, Coleman J, Kreissig I, Richard G, Chang S, Wilcox LM: The perfluorocarbon gases in the treatment of retinal detachment. Ophthalmology, 90 (1983) 546-551

199. Lobel D, Hale JR, Montgomery DB: A new magnetic technique for the treatment of giant retinal tears. Am J Ophthalmol, 85 (1978) 699-703

200. Lucke K, Foerster MH, Laqua H: Langzeiterfahrungen mit intraokularer Silikon-Füllung. Fortschr Ophthalmol, 84 (1987) 96-98

201. Lucke K, Laqua H, Foerster MH: Long-term results of vitrectomy and silicone oil in 500 cases of complicated retinal detachments. Am J Ophthalmol, 104 (1987) 624-633

202. Lucke K, Reinking U, El-Hifnawi E, Dennin RH, Laqua H: Akute retinale Nekrose. Klin Monats Augenheilkd, 193 (1988) 602-607

203. Lund O-E: Silikonöl als Glaskörperersatz. Ber Dtsch Ophthalmol Ges, 68 (1968) 166-169

204. Machemer R, Aaberg TM, Norton WD: Giant retinal tears. II. Experimental production and management with intravitreal air. Am J Ophthalmol, 68 (1969) 1022-1029

205. Machemer R, Buettner H, Norton EWD, Parel JM: Vitrectomy. A pars plana approach. Trans Am Acad Ophthalmol Otolaryngol, 75 (1971) 813-820

206. Machemer R, Laqua H: Pigment epithelium proliferation in retinal detachment (massive periretinal proliferation). Am J Ophthalmol, 80 (1975) 1-23

207. Machemer R, Allen AW: Retinal tears 180 degrees and greater. Management with vitrectomy and intravitreal gas. Arch Ophthalmol, 94 (1976) 1340-1346

208. Machemer R: Massive periretinal proliferation. A logical approach to therapy. Trans Am Ophthalmol Soc, 75 (1977) 556-586

209. Machemer R, Laqua H: A logical approach to the treatment of massive periretinal proliferation. Ophthalmology, 85 (1978) 584-593

210. Machemer R: Vitrectomy: A pars plana approach. Grune & Stratton, New York, (1975)

211. Machemer R, McCuen BW II, de Juan E: Relaxing retinotomies and retinectomies. Am J Ophthalmol, 102 (1986) 7-12

212. Manschot WA: Intravitreal silicone injection. Adv Ophthalmol, 36 (1978) 197-207

213. Margherio RR, Schepens CL: Macular breaks. 2. Management. Am J Ophthalmol, 74 (1972) 233-240

214. May DR, Peyman GA Endophthalmitis after vitrectomy. Am J Ophthalmol, 81 (1876) 520-521

215. McCuen BW II, Landers MB III, Machemer R: The use of silicone oil following failed vitrectomy for retinal detachment with advanced proliferative vitreoretinopathy. Ophthalmology, 92 (1985) 1029-1034

216. McCuen BW II, Hida T, Sheta SM, Isbey EK, Hahn DK, Hickingbotham D: Experimental transvitreal cyanoacrylate retinopexy. Am J Ophthalmol, 102 (1986) 199-207

217. McCuen BW II, Rinkoff JS Silicone oil for progressive anterior ocular neovascularization after failed diabetic vitrectomy. Arch Ophthalmol, 107 (1989) 677-682

218. McLean EB, Norton EWD: Use of intraocular air and sulfur hexafluoride gas in the repair of selected retinal detachments. Mod Probl Ophthal, 12 (1974) 428-435

219. McLeod D: Silicone oil injection during closed microsurgery for diabetic retinal detachment. Graefe's Arch Clin Exp Ophthalmol, 224 (1986) 55-59

220. Mehdorn E, Lucke K, Steinmetz M: Transscleral cyclocoagulation with the neodymium:YAG-cw laser: comparison of anterior and posterior coagulation. Lasers Light Opthalmol (1990) (in press)

221. Meredith T, Lindsey DT, Edelhauser HF, Goldman A: Electroretinographic studies following vitrectomy and intraocular silicone injection. Br J Ophthalmol, 69 (1985) 254-260

222. Mester U, Kroll P, Völker B, Kreissig I: Intraocular SF6-gas applications: Treatment of retinal detachments caused by holes at the posterior pole. Ophthalmologica, 180 (1983) 151-155

223. Meyer-Schwickerath G: Lichtkoagulation. Enke, Stuttgart (1959)

224. Meyer-Schwickerath G: Macular holes and retinal detachment. In: New and controversial aspects of retinal detachment, Hoeber, New York (1968) 443-447

225. Meyer-Schwickerath G, Lund OE, Höpping W: Six years experienc e with silicone injections into the vitreous cavity. Trans New Orleans Acad Ophthalmol (1969)

226. Michels RG: Vitrectomy for complications of diabetic retinopathy. Arch Ophthalmol, 96 (1978) 237-246

227. Michels RG: Vitreous surgery. Mosby, St. Louis, (1981)

228. Michels RG, Rice TA, Blankenship G: Surgical techniques for selected giant retinal tears. Retina, 3 (1983) 139-145

229. Michels RG: Vitrectomy for macular pucker. Ophthalmology, 91 (1984) 1384-1388

230. Miller B, Miller H, Ryan S: Experimental retinal hole: an in vivo model for cellular proliferation. Invest Ophthalmol Vis Sci, 26 (1985) 59-65

231. Miller B, Miller H, Ryan SJ: Experimental epiretinal proliferation induced by intravitreal red blood cells. Am J Ophthalmol, 102 (1986) 188-195

232. Miller B, Miller H, Patterson R, Ryan S: Retinal wound healing. Arch Ophthalmol, 104 (1986) 281-285

233. Miller B, Miller H, Patterson R, Ryan S: Effect of the vitreous on retinal wound healing. Graefe's Arch Clin Exp Ophthalmol, 224 (1986) 576-579

234. Miyake Y: A simplified method of treating retinal detachment with macular hole. Am J Ophthalmol, 97 (1984) 243-245

235. Miyamoto K, Refojo MF, Tolentino FI, Fournier GA, Albert DM: Perfluoroether liquid as a long-term vitreous subsitute. An experimental study. Retina, 4 (1984) 264-268

236. Miyamoto K, Refojo MF, Tolentino FI, Fournier GA, Albert DM: Fluorinated oils as experimental vitreous substitutes. Arch Ophthalmol, 104 (1986) 1053-1056

237. Momirov D, van Lith GHM, Živojnović R: Electroretinogram and electrooculogram of eyes with intravitreously injected silicone oil. Ophthalmologica, 186 (1983) 183-188

238. Moreau PG: Implant into the vitreous using silicone for detachment of the retina. Trans Ophthalmol Soc UK, 84 (1964) 167-171

239. Mukai N, Lee PF, Schepens CL: Intravitreous injection of silicone An experimental study. Ann Ophthalmol, 4 (1972) 273-287

240. Mukai N, Lee PF, Oguri M, Schepens CL: A long-term evaluation of silicone retinopathy in monkeys. Can J Ophthalmol, 10 (1975) 391-402

241. Müller-Jensen K, Köhler H: Versuche eines Glaskörperersatzes durch Polyacrylamid. Ber Dtsch Ophthalmol Ges, 68 (1968) 181-184

242. Ni C, Wang WJ, Albert DM, Schepens CL: Intravitreous silicone injection. Histopathologic findings in a human eye after 12 years. Arch Ophthalmol, 101 (1983) 1399-1401

243. Norton EWD, Aaberg TM, Fung W, Curtin VT: Giant retinal tears I. Clinical management with intravitreal air. Am J Ophthalmol, 68 (1969) 1011-1021

244. O'Connor GR: Calcific band keratopathy. Trans Am Ophthalmol Soc, 70 (1969) 58-81

245. O'Grady GE, Parel J-M, Lee W, Flynn HW, Olsen KR, Blankenship G, Clarkson JG: Hypodermic stainless steel tacks and companion inserter designed for peripheral fixation of retina. Arch Ophthalmol, 106 (1988) 271-275

246. Ober RR, Blanks JC, Ogden TE, Pickford M, Minckler DS, Ryan SJ: Experimental retinal tolerance to liquid silicone. Retina, 3 (1983) 77-85

247. Ohm J: Über die Behandlung der Netzhautablösung durch operative Entleerung der subretinalen Flüssigkeit und Einspritzung von Luft in den Glaskörper. Graefe's Arch Clin Exp Ophthalmol, 79 (1911) 442-450

248. Okun E: Therapy of retinal detachment complicated by massive pre-retinal fibroplasia. Ber Dtsch Ophthalmol Ges, 68 (1968) 150-154

249. Okun E: The current status of silicone oil (analysis of long term successes) In: Advances in vitreous surgery, Thomas, Springfield (1976) 518-522

250. Olson RJ: Air and the corneal endothelium. An in vivo specular microscopy in cats. Arch Ophthalmol, 98 (1980) 1283-1284

251. Parmley VC, Barishak YR, Howes EL, Crawford JB: Foreign-body giant cell reaction to liquid silicone. Am J Ophthalmol, 101 (1986) 680-683

252. Paufique L, Morean PG cited in Liesenhoff 1968 Ann Ocul, 186 (1953) 873-875

253. Petersen J, Ritzau-Tondrow U, Vogel M: Fluor-Silikonöl schwerer als Wasser: ein neues Hilfsmittel der vitreo-retinalen Chirurgie. Klin Monats Augenheilkd, 189 (1986) 228-232

254. Petersen J, Ritzau-Tondrow, U: Chronisches Glaukom nach Silikonölimplantation: Zwei Öle verschiedener Viskosität im Vergleich. Fortschr Ophthalmol 85 (1988) 632-634

255. Petersen J: The physical and surgical aspects of silicone oil in the vitreous cavity. Graefe's Arch Clin Exp Ophthalmol, 225 (1988) 452-456

256. Peyman GA, Vygantas CM, Bennett TO, Vygantas AM, Brubaker S: Octafluorocyclobutane in vitreous and aqueous humor replacement. Arch Ophthalmol, 93 (1975) 514-517

257. Peyman GA, Huamonte FU, Goldberg MF, Sanders DR, Nagpal KC, Raichand M: Four hundred consecutive pars plana vitrectomies with the vitrophage. Arch Ophthalmol, 96 (1978) 45-54

258. Peyman GA, Rednam KRV, Seetner AA: Retinal microincarceration with penetrating diathermy in the management of giant retinal tears. Arch Ophthalmol, 102 (1984) 562-565

259. Polemann G, Froitzheim G: Tierexperimentelle Untersuchungen zur biologischen Verträglichkeit von Silikonen. Arzneimittelforschung, 3 (1953) 457-461

260. Rachal WF, Burton TC: Changing concepts of failures after retinal detachment surgery. Arch Ophthalmol, 97 (1979) 480-483

261. Ratner CM, Michels RG, Auer C, Rice TA: Pars plana vitrectomy for complicated retinal detachments. Ophthalmology, 90 (1983) 1323-1327

262. Refojo FM, Leong F, Chung H, Ueno N, Nemiroff B, Tolentino FI: Extraction of retinol and cholesterol by intraocular silicone oils. Ophthalmology, 95 (1988) 614-618

263. Rentsch FJ, Atzler P, Liesenhoff H: Histologische und elektronenmikroskopische Untersuchungen an einem menschlichen Auge nach mehrjähriger intravitrealer Silikonölimplantation. Ber Dtsch Ophthalmol Ges, 75 (1977) 70-74

264. Rice TA, Michels RG: Long-term anatomic and functional results of vitrectomy for diabetic retinopathy. Am J Ophthalmol, 90 (1980) 297-303

265. Rice TA, Michels RG, Rice EF: Vitrectomy for diabetic traction detachment involving the macula. Am J Ophthalmol, 95 (1983) 22-33

266. Riedel KG, Gabel V-P, Neubauer L, Kampik A, Lund O-E: Intravitreal silicone injection: complications and treatment of 415 consecutive patients. Graefe's Arch Clin Exp Ophthalmol, 228 (1990) 19-23

267. Rinkoff JS, de Juan E, McCuen BW II: Silicone oil for retinal detachment with advanced proliferative vitreoretinopathy following failed vitrectomy for proliferative diabetic retinopathy. Am J Ophthalmol, 101 (1986) 181-186

268. Rosengren B: Über die Behandlung der Netzhautablösung mittelst Diathermie und Luft-Injektion in den Glaskörper. Acta Ophthalmol (Copenh), 16 (1938) 3-42

269. Ryan SJ: The pathophysiology of proliferative vitreoretinopathy in its management. Am J Ophthalmol, 100 (1985) 188-193

270. Ryan SJ: Proliferative vitreoretinopathy – the Silicone Study Group. Am J Ophthalmol, 99 (1985) 593-595

271. Schatz H, McDonald HR: Treatment of sensory retinal detachment associated with optic nerve pit or coloboma. Ophthalmology, 95 (1988) 178-186

272. Schepens CL: Scleral buckling with circling element. Trans Am Acad Ophthalmol Otolaryngol, 68 (1964) 959-966

273. Schepens CL, Freeman HM: Current management of giant retinal breaks. Trans Am Acad Ophthalmol Otolaryngol, 71 (1967) 474 -487

274. Schepens CL: A new ophthalmoscope demonstration. Trans Am Acad Ophthalmol Otolaryngol, 51 (1947) 298-304

275. Schepens CL: Retinal detachment and allied diseases. Saunders, Philadelphia, (1983)

276. Scott JD: A new approach to the vitreous base. Mod Probl Ophthal, 12 (1974) 407-410

277. Scott JD: Macular holes and retinal detachment. Trans Ophthalmol Soc UK, 94 (1974) 319-324

278. Scott JD: A rationale for the use of liquid silicone. Trans Ophthalmol Soc UK, 97 (1977) 235-237

279. Scott JD: Lens epthelial proliferation in retinal detachment. Trans Ophthalmol Soc UK, 102 (1982) 385-389

280. Sebestyen JG: Fibrinoid syndrome: a severe complication of vitreous surgery in diabetics. Ann Ophthalmol, 14 (1982) 853-856

281. Sell C, McCuen BW II, Landers MB III, Machemer R: Long-term results of successful vitrectomy with silicone oil for advanced proliferative vitreoretinopathy. Am J Ophthalmol, 103 (1987) 24-28

282. Shafer DM: The treatment of retinal detachment by vitreous implant. Trans Am Acad Ophthalmol Otolaryngol, 61 (1957) 194-200

283. Sheta SM, Hida T, McCuen BW II: Experimental transvitreal cyanoacrylate retinopexy through silicone oil. Am J Ophthalmol, 102 (1986) 717-722

284. Sheta SM, Hida TH, McCuen BW II: Cyanoacrylate tissue adhesive in the management of recurrent retinal detachment caused by macular hole. Am J Ophthalmol, 109 (1990) 28-32

285. Shields CL, Eagle RC: Pseudo-Schnabel's cavernous degeneration of the optic nerve secondary to intraocular silicone oil. Arch Ophthalmol, 107 (1989) 714-717

286. Shugar JK, de Juan E, McCuen BW II, Tiedemann J, Landers MB III: Ultrasonic examination of the silicone filled eye: theoretical and practical considerations. Graefe's Arch Clin Exp Ophthalmol, 224 (1986) 361-367

287. Siam AL: Décollement de la rétina causé par un trou maculaire. Bull Mem Soc Fr Ophthalmol, 91 (1979) 150-156

288. Skorpik Ch, Gnad HD, Menapace R, Paroussis P: Erste Erfahrungen mit primärer Silikonfüllung des Glaskörperraumes bei komplizierten Augenverletzungen. Klin Monats Augenheilkd, 191 (1987) 113-115

289. Skorpik C, Menapace R, Gnad HD, Paroussis P: Silicone oil implantation in penetrating injuries complicated by PVR. Retina, 9 (1989) 8-14

290. Spitznas M: A binocular indirect ophthalmomicroscope (BIOM) for non-contact wide-angle vitreous surgery. Graefe's Arch Clin Exp Ophthalmol, 225 (1987) 13-15

291. Stefánsson E, Landers MB III, Wolbarsht ML: Vitrectomy, lensectomy and ocular oxygenation. Retina, 2 (1982) 159-166

292. Stefánsson E, Tiedemann JS: Optics of the eye with air or silicone. Retina, 8 (1988) 10-19

293. Stefánsson E, Anderson MM, Landers MB III, Tiedemann JS, McCuen BW II: Refractive changes from use of silicone oil in vitreous surgery. Retina, 8 (1988) 20-23

294. Sternberg P, Machemer R: Results of conventional vitreous surgery for proliferative vitreoretinopathy. Am J Ophthalmol, 100 (1985) 141-146

295. Sternberg P, Han DP, Yeo JH, Barr CC, Lewis H, Williams GA, Mieler WF: Photocoagulation to prevent retinal detachment in acute retinal necrosis. Ophthalmology, 95 (1988) 1389-1393

296. Stone W: Alloplasty in surgery of the eye. N Engl J Med, 258 (1958) 486-491

297. Sugar HS, Okamura ID: Ocular findings six years after intravitreal silicone injection. Arch Ophthalmol, 94 (1976) 612-615

298. Tano Y, Chandler D, Machemer R: Treatment of intraocular proliferation with intravitreal injection of triamcinolone acetonide. Am J Ophthalmol, 90 (1980) 810-816

299. Tavakolian U, Wollensak J: Ergebnisse von Silikonölinjektionen in den verschiedenen Stadien der proliferativen Vitreoretinopathie. Klin Monats Augenheilkd, 186 (1985) 268-271

300. Thaler A, Lessel MR, Gnad H, Heilig P: The influence of intravitreally injected silicone oil on electrophysiological potentials of the eye. Doc Ophthalmol Proc, 62 (1986) 41-46

301. The Retina Society Terminology Committee: The classification of retinal detachment with proliferative vitreoretinopathy. Ophthalmology, 90 (1983) 121-125

302. Theodossiadis G: Treatment of retinal detachment arising from macular holes. Mod Probl Ophthal, 12 (1974) 322-329

303. Thompson JT, Auer CL, de Bustros S, Michels RG, Rice TA, Glaser BM: Prognostic indicators of success and failure in vitrectomy for diabetic retinopathy. Ophthalmology, 93 (1986) 290-295

304. Thompson JT, Bustros S, Michels G, Rice TA: Results and prognostic factors in vitrectomy for diabetic traction retinal detachment of the macula. Arch Ophthalmol, 105 (1987) 497-502

305. Thompson JT, Bustros S, Michels RG, Rice TA: Results and prognostic factors in vitrectomy for diabetic traction-rhegmatogenous retinal detachment. Arch Ophthalmol, 105 (1987) 503-507

306. Tolentino FI, Schepens CL, Freeman HM: Massive preretinal retraction. Arch Ophthalmol, 78 (1967) 16-20

307. Tolentino FI, Cajita VN, Chung H, Acosta J, Freeman HM, Refojo MF: High density fluorosilicone oil in vitreous surgery. In: Proliferative vitreoretinopathie (PVR). Springer, Berlin Heidelberg New York (1988) 177-180

308. Topping M, Abrams GW, Machemer R: Experimental double-perforating injury of the posterior segment in rabbit eyes. Arch Ophthalmol, 97 (1979) 735-742

309. Usui M, Hamasaki S, Takano S, Matsuo H: A new surgical technique for the treatment of giant tear: transvitreoretinal fixation. Jpn J Ophthalmol, 23 (1979) 206-215

310. van Horn DL, Edelhauser AF, Aaberg TM: In vivo effects of air and sulfur hexafluoride gas on rabbit corneal endothelium. Invest Ophthalmol Vis Sci, 11 (1972) 1028-1036

311. Watzke RC: Silicone retinopoesis for retinal detachment. Arch Ophthalmol, 77 (1967) 185-196

312. Watzke RC: Silicone retinopiesis for retinal detachment. A pathological report. Surv Ophthalmol, 12 (1967) 333-337

313. Wessing A, Spitznas M, Palomar A: Management of retinal detachments due to giant tears. Graefe's Arch Clin Exp Ophthalmol, 192 (1974) 277-284

314. Widder W: Hyaluronsäure als Glaskörperimplantat bei Netzhautablösungen. Albrecht von Graefe's Arch Ophthalmol, 162 (1960) 416-429

315. Wiedemann P, Lemmen K, Schmiedl R, Heimann K: Intraocular daunorubicin for the treatment and prophylaxis of traumatic proliferative vitreoretinopathy. Am J Ophthalmol, 104 (1987) 10-14

316. Wiedemann P, Wiedemann R, Lemmen K, Heimann K: Intraokulares Daunomycin zur Behandlung der proliferativen Vitreoretinopathie. 85. Meeting of the Deutsche Ophthalmolgische Gesellschaft, Heidelberg (1987) Sept 20 – 23

317. Wilflingseder P, Propst A, Mikuz G Constrictive fibrosis following silicone implants in mammary augmentation. Chir plast, 2 (1974) 215-229

318. Wintsch W, Smahel J, Clodius L Local and regional lymph node response to ruptured gel-filled mammary prostheses. Br J Plast Surg, 41 (1978) 349-352

319. Yamauchi A: Preparation and properties of PVA hydrogel and its behaviour in the vitreous body of albino rabbit. International polymer conference, Kyoto (1984) August 20-24

320. Yamauchi A: Synthetic vitreous body. Research institute for polymers and textiles, (1986)

321. Yeo JH, Glaser BM, Michels RG: Silicone oil in the treatment of complicated retinal detachments. Ophthalmology, 94 (1987) 1109-1113

322. Zhu Z-R, Sorgente N, Blanks JC, Ogden TE, Ryan SJ: Cellular proliferation induced by subretinal injection of vitreous in the rabbit. Arch Ophthalmol, 106 (1988) 406-411

323. Zilis JD, McCuen BW II, de Juan E Jr, Stefànsson E, Machemer R: Results of silicone oil removal in advanced proliferative vitreoretinopathy. Am J Ophthalmol, 108 (1989) 15-21

324. Živojnović R, Mertens DAE, Baarsma GS: Das flüssige Silikon in der Amotiochirurgie. Klin Monats Augenheilkd, 179 (1981) 17-22

325. Živojnović R, Mertens DAE, Peperkamp E: Das flüssige Silikon in der Amotiochirurgie (II). Bericht über 280 Fälle – weitere Entwicklung der Technik. Klin Monats Augenheilkd, 181 (1982) 444-452

326. Živojnović R: Silicone oil in vitreoretinal surgery. Nijhoff/Junk, Dordrecht (1987)

# Appendix

**Table A.** Absolute anatomic and functional results (early group)

| Diagnosis | *n* | Successes at the end of follow-up | | | | | | Follow-up (months) |
|---|---|---|---|---|---|---|---|---|
| | | Anatomical | | Visual | | Visual acuity ≥1/50 | | |
| | | *n* | % | *n* | % | *n* | % | |
| All diagnoses | 184 | 127 | 69.0 | 98 | 53.3 | 102 | 55.4 | 28.7 |
| ≥ 6 mos. follow-up | 164 | 115 | 70.1 | 91 | 55.5 | 96 | 58.5 | 31.9 |
| PVR, total | 96 | 55 | 57.3 | 40 | 41.7 | 44 | 45.8 | 28.5 |
| without perforating injury | 76 | 46 | 60.5 | 32 | 42.1 | 37 | 48.7 | 29.2 |
| with perforating injury | 20 | 9 | 45.0 | 8 | 40.0 | 7 | 35.0 | 26.0 |
| with giant tears | 15 | 7 | 46.7 | 3 | 20.0 | 5 | 33.3 | 25.5 |
| with posterior holes | 10 | 6 | 60.0 | 3 | 30.0 | 3 | 30.0 | 29.3 |
| PVR,uncomplicated | 55 | 33 | 60.0 | 26 | 47.3 | 29 | 52.7 | 29.9 |
| Stage C | 13 | 8 | 61.5 | 5 | 38.5 | 7 | 53.8 | 22.4 |
| Stage C1 | 4 | 3 | 75.0 | 2 | 50.0 | 3 | 75.0 | 9.8 |
| Stage C2 | 4 | 3 | 75.0 | 3 | 75.0 | 3 | 75.0 | 19.5 |
| Stage C3 | 5 | 2 | 40.0 | 0 | 0.0 | 1 | 20.0 | 34.8 |
| Stage D | 42 | 25 | 59.5 | 21 | 50.0 | 22 | 52.4 | 32.2 |
| Stage D1 | 13 | 10 | 76.9 | 7 | 53.8 | 8 | 61.5 | 38.5 |
| Stage D2 | 22 | 11 | 50.0 | 10 | 45.5 | 11 | 50.0 | 31.1 |
| Stage D3 | 7 | 4 | 57.1 | 4 | 57.1 | 3 | 42.9 | 23.9 |
| Giant tears, total | 49 | 39 | 79.6 | 27 | 55.1 | 29 | 59.2 | 26.6 |
| uncomplicated | 30 | 28 | 93.3 | 20 | 66.7 | 20 | 66.7 | 26.5 |
| Posterior holes, total | 37 | 28 | 75.7 | 22 | 59.5 | 24 | 64.9 | 27.6 |
| uncomplicated | 26 | 22 | 84.6 | 19 | 73.1 | 21 | 80.8 | 26.5 |
| MH. uncomplicated | 12 | 12 | 00.0 | 10 | 83.3 | 11 | 91.7 | 21.4 |
| PDR, total | 24 | 17 | 70.8 | 14 | 58.3 | 12 | 50.0 | 34.2 |
| with detachment | 17 | 10 | 58.8 | 8 | 47.1 | 6 | 35.3 | 36.9 |
| without detachment | 7 | 7 | 00.0 | 6 | 85.7 | 6 | 85.7 | 27.6 |
| Perforating injury, total | 26 | 14 | 53.8 | 13 | 50.0 | 12 | 46.2 | 25.3 |

PVR, proliferative vitreoretinopathy; MH, macular hole; PDR, proliferative diabetic retinopathy

**Table B.** Anatomic and functional successes after 6 and 24 months by life table analysis[1] (early group)

| Diagnosis | n | Anatomical | | Visual | | Visual acuity ≥1/50 | |
|---|---|---|---|---|---|---|---|
| | | 6 | 24 | 6 | 24 | 6 | 24 |
| All diagnoses | 184 | 75 | 67 | 67 | 52 | 60 | 54 |
| ≥ 6 mos. follow-up | 164 | 77 | 69 | 71 | 55 | 64 | 57 |
| PVR, total | 96 | 66 | 53 | 60 | 40 | 48 | 43 |
| without perforating injury | 76 | 67 | 57 | 56 | 43 | 51 | 46 |
| with perforating injury | 20 | 64 | 34 | 75 | 25 | 25 | 25 |
| with giant tears | 15 | 53 | 46 | 53 | 25 | 33 | 33 |
| with posterior holes | 10 | 70 | 52 | 50 | 26 | 30 | 30 |
| PVR, uncomplicated | 55 | 67 | 57 | 62 | 48 | 56 | 49 |
| Stage C | 13 | 61 | 61 | 46 | 35 | 62 | 50 |
| Stage C1 | 4 | 75 | 75 | 50 | 50 | 75 | 75 |
| Stage C2 | 4 | 75 | 75 | 71 | 71 | 75 | 75 |
| Stage C3 | 5 | 40 | 40 | 0 | 0 | 40 | 20 |
| Stage D | 42 | 69 | 57 | 67 | 52 | 55 | 49 |
| Stage D1 | 13 | 77 | 77 | 69 | 61 | 54 | 54 |
| Stage D2 | 22 | 63 | 45 | 64 | 47 | 55 | 49 |
| Stage D3 | 7 | 71 | 36 | 71 | 48 | 57 | 29 |
| Giant tears, total | 49 | 82 | 79 | 69 | 57 | 65 | 60 |
| uncomplicated | 30 | 93 | 93 | 73 | 69 | 77 | 68 |
| Posterior holes, total | 37 | 81 | 73 | 70 | 55 | 65 | 65 |
| uncomplicated | 26 | 88 | 83 | 81 | 70 | 81 | 81 |
| MH uncomplicated | 12 | 100 | 100 | 83 | 83 | 92 | 92 |
| PDR,total | 24 | 75 | 70 | 71 | 56 | 67 | 49 |
| with detachment | 17 | 64 | 57 | 58 | 45 | 53 | 35 |
| without detachment | 7 | 100 | 100 | 100 | 83 | 100 | 83 |
| Perforating injury, total | 26 | 69 | 46 | 77 | 38 | 46 | 46 |

PVR, proliferative vitreoretinopathy; MH, macular hole; PDR, proliferative diabetic retinopathy

[1]Values constitute cumulative proportions

**Table C.** Absolute anatomic and functional results (late group)

| Diagnosis | *n* | Successes at the end of follow-up | | | | | | Follow-up (months) |
|---|---|---|---|---|---|---|---|---|
| | | Anatomical | | Visual | | Visual acuity ≥1/50 | | |
| | | *n* | % | *n* | % | *n* | % | |
| All diagnoses | 299 | 223 | 74.6 | 185 | 61.9 | 211 | 70.6 | 17.4 |
| ≥ 6 mos. follow-up | 236 | 178 | 75.4 | 157 | 66.5 | 174 | 73.7 | 21.4 |
| PVR, total | 130 | 97 | 74.6 | 91 | 70.0 | 101 | 77.7 | 17.7 |
| without perforating injury | 105 | 82 | 78.1 | 75 | 71.4 | 84 | 80.0 | 18.6 |
| with perforating injury | 25 | 15 | 60.0 | 16 | 64.0 | 17 | 68.0 | 13.8 |
| with giant tears | 5 | 4 | 80.0 | 3 | 60.0 | 5 | 100.0 | 14.0 |
| with posterior holes | 13 | 10 | 76.9 | 9 | 69.2 | 11 | 84.6 | 21.4 |
| PVR, uncomplicated | 89 | 70 | 78.7 | 65 | 73.0 | 71 | 79.8 | 18.0 |
| Stage C | 29 | 24 | 82.8 | 18 | 62.1 | 24 | 82.8 | 18.9 |
| Stage C1 | 4 | 4 | 100.0 | 4 | 100.0 | 4 | 100.0 | 37.8 |
| Stage C2 | 18 | 14 | 77.8 | 11 | 61.1 | 14 | 77.8 | 16.4 |
| Stage C3 | 7 | 6 | 85.7 | 3 | 42.9 | 6 | 85.7 | 14.6 |
| Stage D | 60 | 46 | 76.7 | 47 | 78.3 | 47 | 78.3 | 17.6 |
| Stage D1 | 14 | 14 | 100.0 | 14 | 100.0 | 14 | 100.0 | 22.4 |
| Stage D2 | 36 | 24 | 66.7 | 25 | 69.4 | 25 | 69.4 | 15.7 |
| Stage D3 | 10 | 8 | 80.0 | 8 | 80.0 | 8 | 80.0 | 17.7 |
| Giant tears, total | 21 | 19 | 90.5 | 16 | 76.2 | 20 | 95.2 | 18.3 |
| uncomplicated | 15 | 14 | 93.3 | 12 | 80.0 | 14 | 93.3 | 20.8 |
| Posterior holes, total | 34 | 28 | 82.4 | 24 | 70.6 | 27 | 79.4 | 19.2 |
| uncomplicated | 21 | 18 | 85.7 | 15 | 71.4 | 16 | 76.2 | 17.8 |
| MH, uncomplicated | 9 | 8 | 88.9 | 5 | 55.6 | 7 | 77.8 | 17.6 |
| PDR, total | 112 | 79 | 70.5 | 59 | 52.7 | 70 | 62.5 | 16.3 |
| with detachment | 107 | 76 | 71.0 | 56 | 52.3 | 67 | 62.6 | 16.1 |
| without detachment | 5 | 3 | 60.0 | 3 | 60.0 | 3 | 60.0 | 20.2 |
| Perforating injury, total | 35 | 23 | 65.7 | 22 | 62.9 | 23 | 65.7 | 14.9 |

PVR, proliferative vitreoretinopathy; MH, macular hole; PDR, proliferative diabetic retinopathy

**Table D.** Anatomic and functional successes after 6 and 24 months by life table analysis[1] (late group)

| Diagnosis | *n* | Anatomical | | Visual | | Visual acuity ≥1/50 | |
|---|---|---|---|---|---|---|---|
| | | 6 | 24 | 6 | 24 | 6 | 24 |
| All diagnoses | 299 | 76 | 72 | 64 | 60 | 72 | 66 |
| ≥ 6 mos. follow-up | 236 | 79 | 74 | 70 | 66 | 77 | 71 |
| PVR, total | 130 | 77 | 72 | 72 | 69 | 78 | 72 |
| without perforating injury | 105 | 79 | 76 | 75 | 70 | 82 | 76 |
| with perforating injury | 25 | 65 | 53 | 61 | 61 | 61 | 55 |
| with giant tears | 5 | 78 | 78 | 57 | 57 | 78 | 78 |
| with posterior holes | 13 | 76 | 76 | 68 | 68 | 85 | 85 |
| PVR, uncomplicated | 89 | 80 | 76 | 77 | 72 | 82 | 74 |
| Stage C | 29 | 85 | 79 | 65 | 60 | 90 | 73 |
| Stage C1 | 4 | 100 | 100 | 100 | 100 | 100 | 100 |
| Stage C2 | 18 | 83 | 73 | 66 | 58 | 89 | 61 |
| Stage C3 | 7 | 83 | 83 | 43 | 43 | 86 | 86 |
| Stage D | 60 | 78 | 74 | 83 | 78 | 78 | 75 |
| Stage D1 | 14 | 100 | 100 | 100 | 100 | 100 | 100 |
| Stage D2 | 36 | 68 | 63 | 74 | 69 | 72 | 66 |
| Stage D3 | 10 | 78 | 78 | 90 | 75 | 70 | 70 |
| Giant tears, total | 21 | 90 | 90 | 74 | 74 | 90 | 90 |
| uncomplicated | 15 | 93 | 93 | 79 | 79 | 93 | 93 |
| Posterior holes, total | 34 | 85 | 81 | 73 | 69 | 85 | 81 |
| uncomplicated | 21 | 90 | 83 | 76 | 70 | 86 | 78 |
| MH, uncomplicated | 9 | 89 | 89 | 67 | 52 | 89 | 69 |
| PDR, total | 112 | 72 | 68 | 56 | 50 | 65 | 58 |
| with detachment | 107 | 73 | 70 | 55 | 51 | 65 | 60 |
| without detachment | 5 | 60 | 60 | 80 | 48 | 60 | 36 |
| Perforating injury, total | 35 | 70 | 61 | 61 | 61 | 61 | 56 |

PVR, proliferative vitreoretinopathy; MH, macular hole; PDR, proliferative diabetic retinopathy

[1]Values constitute cumulative proportions

# Subject Index